Cardiovascular
Case Studies
in Primary Care
by
Beverley Cox
RGN BSc MSc

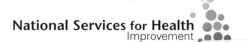

National Services for Health
Improvement

Cardiovascular Case Studies in Primary Care

by Beverley Cox RGN BSc MSc

Published in the UK by:

National Services for Health Improvement

Nucleus@The Bridge

London Science and Business Park

Brunel Way, Dartford DA1 5GA

Copyright 2010 National Services for Health Improvement.

Printed in the UK by Nuffield Press Ltd.

ISBN 978-0-9560921-4-4

About the author

Bev Cox RGN BSc MSc

Bev trained at St George's Hospital, London and qualified in 1982. By 1984 she had moved into general practice, where she has remained ever since. As well as working as a nurse practitioner at Walsgrave Health Centre in Coventry for 3.5 days a week, she is also a Clinical Lecturer for Cardiovascular Disease, Cardio-respiratory disease, Diabetes and Smoking Cessation at Education for Health in Warwick, where she writes, develops and delivers education for GPs, nurses and pharmacists. Areas of particular clinical interest include hypertension, lipid management, assessing and managing cardiovascular risk, heart failure, asthma, COPD and diabetes, and Bev has been involved in the development of the diabetes guidelines from NICE.

She has a BSc in Professional Nursing Studies and an MSc in Respiratory Care. She has been a qualified independent and supplementary nurse prescriber since 2003 and has been a speaker at national prescribing conferences.

Bev is a visiting lecturer for Imperial College London's MSc in Preventive Cardiology and has been a Special Visiting Lecturer at Coventry University for several years, teaching coronary heart disease, respiratory disease and ethics. Up until 2006 she was the Nurse Representative on the Professional Executive Committee of Coventry Teaching PCT, which gave her a fascinating insight into the politics of modern healthcare.

Additionally, she sits on the Editorial Boards of the *'British Journal of Primary Care Nursing'* and *'Practice Nursing'* and is a member of the Cardiovascular Nurse Leaders Network, a sub-group of the Primary Care Cardiovascular Society. The CVNL group assisted the Department of Health with the development of the Vascular Screening Programme, now known as NHS

Health Checks. Bev writes regularly for the nursing press and has published two books on cardiovascular disease (*Vital CHD* and this book, *Cardiovascular Case Studies in Primary Care*). She has also written the *'Simply Lipids'* handbook for Education for Health, and *'Simply Risk'*.

Another interest is the concept of developing patient-focused consultations using cognitive behavioural therapy. Her dissertation for her MSc asked the question 'What do patients want from their consultations?' and argued that the quality of patient/clinician communication in the consultation is a key aspect of patient-centred care.

beverley.cox@nhs.net
Walsgrave Health Centre
50 Hall Lane
Coventry
CV2 2SW

Contents

Introduction

Cardiovascular disease (CVD) has been a key target area for clinicians working in primary care for the past decade or more. From the publication of the first National Service Framework for Coronary Heart Disease in 2000 to the 'Putting Prevention First' programme in 2008, which led to the initiation of the NHS Health Checks aimed at identifying those at higher risk of cardiovascular disease, primary care has been at the forefront of the battle against CVD. The introduction of the new General Medical Services (nGMS) contract in 2004 aimed to improve the delivery of evidence-based patient care, notably for long term conditions (LTCs) such as CVD. Managing LTCs takes up a large proportion of NHS resources (DH 2005a) and much of this care is delivered by general practitioners and practice nursing staff (DH 2004b), so the contract was a significant move towards delivering a quality driven general practice service. The contract allocates points for the provision of evidence-based, quality care; the points have a monetary value and the more points that are gained, the greater the amount of money that is paid to the practice. This is the first time that general practitioners have been paid directly for the quality of the work that they are doing in terms of clinical care provision, improved record keeping, data collection, faster access and patient satisfaction.

The number of guidelines coming out from the Department of Health and other bodies such as the National Institute of Health and Clinical Excellence (NICE) continues unabated. This can make it difficult for clinicians to keep up to date with recent developments. One way in which people have been shown to learn is through case study examples, which may be easier to remember. The following cases are based on actual patients seen in practice by the author, although identities have been disguised to protect patient confidentiality and some cases are composites of various patients seen over the years. Evidence changes constantly and so, then, does best practice. We are currently seeing much debate, for instance, around the use of aspirin in primary and secondary prevention of CVD. Although these case studies were treated using examples of best practice at the time of writing, it is important to remain mindful of new developments which are constantly on the horizon. However, the focus of this book is on the implementation of evidence-based care for patients with CVD in a general practice setting. The author has worked in general practice since 1984 and continues to do so to this day. The cases are a few examples of the rich tapestry of her clinical practice as a nurse practitioner.

Typical cardiac chest pain presentation and management, to include risk factors, history taking, examination, signs and symptoms, immediate and long term management.

Case study 1: Mr Jenkins

Mr Jenkins is a 49 year old miner who presented at the surgery for a hypertension review. He was taking atenolol 50mg and ramipril 2.5mg daily for this. His blood pressure was well controlled and today was noted to be 132/83. However, he commented that he had been suffering from occasional central chest pains over the past 2-3 months and wondered whether it was worth mentioning them as his father had died after his third heart attack at the age of 72.

Mr Jenkins is overweight, which he puts down to a beer belly as he enjoys several pints at his social club with his work mates. He gave up smoking three months ago as it was costing too much – prior to this he had smoked 20-30 per day, starting at the age of 15 years.

What do you need to know?

Mr Jenkins' history of hypertension is a known risk factor for cardiovascular disease. Other risk factors include his positive family history. Although his blood pressure is well controlled, atenolol is no longer recommended as an option for hypertension management following the findings of the ASCOT trial, as beta blockers do not offer protection against cardiovascular events in people who do not have a history of CVD. In view of the fact that Mr Jenkins is overweight, with a BMI of 33 and a waist measurement of 90cm, he will have an increased risk of metabolic syndrome and type 2 diabetes. Many people have undiagnosed metabolic syndrome and/or diabetes and Mr Jenkins could be one of these people. If so, this is another risk factor for coronary heart disease. Even if he does not have metabolic syndrome or type 2 diabetes, his weight and central obesity will put him at risk of cardiovascular disease.

Definition of metabolic syndrome

Metabolic syndrome is defined as central obesity (waist circumference $\geq$ 94cm for European men and $\geq$ 80cms for European women) and any two of the four factors below:

- ◆ Triglycerides $\geq$ 1.7mmol/L or on treatment for this

- ◆ High Density Lipoprotein Cholesterol (HDL-C) < 1.03mmol/L in men, < 1.29mmol/L in women, or on specific treatment for this

- ◆ BP $\geq$ 130/85 or on treatment for hypertension

- ◆ Fasting Plasma Glucose $\geq$ 5.6mmol/L or diagnosed type 2 diabetes

International Diabetes Federation, 2004

The description of the chest pain is an important diagnostic guide, as a good history can give a clear indication of whether or not cardiovascular disease could be to blame. The PQRST tool can be useful for getting a full history.

Table 1.1: The PQRST Tool	
P:	palliative/provocative
Q:	quality
R:	radiation
S:	severity
T:	timing

Using the PQRST tool, the nurse was able to elicit the following information:

Mr Jenkins explained that the pain came on when he was doing something active but that it would ease off if he rested. He described the pain as a being like a tight band which felt like a heavy weight across the front of his chest but which only lasted a minute or two. On one occasion it moved up into his jaw. On a pain scale of 0 to 10, with 0 being no pain and 10 being unbearable pain, Mr Jenkins thought that it probably scored a 5-6. He only got the pain on exertion and had never had the pain at rest or during the night.

What sort of examination and investigations might be useful?

Mr Jenkins has enough risk factors and a clear enough history to suggest the presence of coronary heart disease. If an acute myocardial infarction was suspected, emergency admission via a 999 call would be indicated. However,

Mr Jenkins has only had occasional episodes of pain lasting for a few minutes, which resolve with rest, so a referral to the Rapid Access Chest Pain (RACP) clinic is appropriate here. In the meantime, bloods can be taken for baseline information such as a full blood count, renal, thyroid and liver function, glucose and lipid levels. An ECG may provide some useful information but should not be regarded as the be-all and end-all of managing chest pain, as a false negative ECG is not uncommon, much as a false positive can also occur.

How and when should you refer on?

A referral to the RACP clinic should mean that Mr Jenkins is seen fairly quickly so that a full assessment of his possible angina is carried out using exercise testing and other investigations as necessary. In the meantime, aspirin 75mg should be started and a GTN spray should be provided, along with instructions on how to use it, should the pain recur.

Table 1.2: Patient information regarding the use of GTN spray

What is GTN for?

GTN (glyceryl trinitrate) in tablet or spray form is used for the immediate relief of chest pain due to angina. The tablets have a short shelf life and should be thrown away eight weeks after opening the bottle. For this reason, the spray is usually prescribed. Although the spray lasts longer, you need to check the expiry date on the bottle. Angina is a pain which is caused by the heart not having enough oxygen. GTN works by opening up the blood vessels which take oxygen to the heart itself. This allows the heart to get more oxygen and should result in the angina pain going away.

What dose should I take?

One or two sprays of GTN should be pumped under the tongue whenever the pain occurs or before doing anything which you know is likely to bring on angina pains. If possible you should sit down before using GTN. After taking it, you should also rest until the pain goes away.

How will I know it is working?

The pain should ease within five minutes. If it has not, you should repeat the dose after five minutes. If it is still not easing after another five minutes, you should take a third dose of GTN. If a third dose has not relieved the pain, you should dial 999 as this could be a sign of a heart attack. If you find that you need to use your GTN more often than usual, you should make an appointment to see your doctor or nurse.

What side effects might I expect and how common are they?

The side-effects of GTN include headaches, dizziness and a flushed face. These tend to wear off after a while and become less common as time goes on.

In the long term, if the diagnosis of angina is confirmed, Mr Jenkins will need further treatment with a statin, possible uptitration of his ACE inhibitor and the introduction of long-term anti-anginal therapy, such as a beta blocker or a calcium channel blocker.

References

Cox, Beverley. Starting on your GTN spray, *British Journal of Primary Care Nursing – Cardiovascular Disease and Diabetes* Volume 5 Issue 3 May-June 2008 Page 148. *www.bjpcn-cardiovascular.com*

Further information

For further information on the management of coronary heart disease, go to:

www.sign.ac.uk/pdf/sign96.pdf

www.escardio.org/knowledge/guidelines/Management_Stable_Angina_Pectoris.htm

Atypical presentations of cardiac chest pain: how the presentation can alter, including how people with diabetes can have silent ischaemia and MI and how others can confuse co-morbidities with CHD.

Case study 2: Joginder

Joginder, a 73 year old Asian lady, had a history of type 2 diabetes, which was diagnosed 12 years ago. Her granddaughter brought her to the surgery one morning because she was complaining of feeling generally unwell. A review of her records showed that her latest HbA1c was 8.2%, her BMI was 32 and her waist measurement was 107cm. Her lipid profile showed a total cholesterol of 5.3, an HDL of 1.0 and triglycerides of 2.2. Her last blood pressure was 152/89, which was average for her.

On examination today, Joginder was pale and clammy and her BP was 94/53. Her temperature was 36.9 and she had a tachycardia of 112 with a regular rhythm. Urinalysis showed glucose +, protein + and nothing else. She complained of feeling slightly nauseous and was very tired. She had 'total body pain' as she described it: aches and pains all over, although nothing specific.

An ECG was requested by the GP. This showed the typical ST elevation associated with an acute myocardial infarction and she was admitted as an emergency in a blue light ambulance.

Joginder's diabetes increases her risk of CVD but her lack of chest pain made her diagnosis easy to miss. People with diabetes are more likely to suffer from a so-called 'silent MI' where the typical central, crushing cheat pain is absent. For that reason we must always maintain a high index of suspicion whenever anyone with a history of diabetes presents with symptoms of acute illness, where an acute cardiovascular event may occur without obvious chest pain

Case study 3: William

William, aged 80, had a history of severe Chronic Obstructive Pulmonary Disease (COPD) with an FEV1 of 29% of the predicted value and an MRC dyspnoea scale score of 3-4. He attended surgery on a crisp autumn morning complaining of a tight chest and requesting some prednisolone and antibiotics for his symptoms, as these usually helped.

William's tight chest had started off about two days ago but had been intermittent. The current tightness had been there since 4 o'clock that morning, however, and he had been using his salbutamol every hour with no relief. He had a chronic smoker's cough but this was no worse than normal. He had not noticed any alteration in his sputum production and was continuing to produce half an egg cupful of grey phlegm per day. The pain was central, did not radiate and had originally eased off if he stopped 'and caught his breath', although he had not been able to get any relief this way since this morning.

William's age, gender and smoking history mean that Coronary Heart Disease (CHD) is a distinct possibility. Although he presented with his own 'ready-made' diagnosis based on his experiences with his COPD, it is important to make an independent assessment of his signs and symptoms. Importantly, William had used the Levine sign (a clenched fist over the centre of the chest, typically used in cases of ischaemic chest pain) when describing his pain and when this was put into context with the other symptoms it seemed reasonable to request further assessment of William's chest symptoms. He was not complaining of feeling sick or clammy or light-headed, however, but he was getting increasingly agitated about not being given his tablets as requested! Some time was spent explaining that there were some elements of his history which made it possible that his heart was causing his symptoms, rather than his lungs on this occasion. However, in view of the fact that the picture was not fully typical of acute coronary syndrome, the healthcare assistant recorded an ECG which showed ST elevation. At this point, William was given GTN, 300mg of aspirin and was admitted to hospital immediately via a 999 call.

Hypertension affects one in five people in the UK and is often managed sub-optimally, despite a range of drug and lifestyle interventions which are known to be useful and effective. We are constantly reminded about the importance of getting people to target with blood pressure treatments but this can be easier said than done. In this chapter we will look at the challenge of getting blood pressure readings down to target levels and we will work through some case studies in order to reach some possible solutions to the difficult problem of achieving the targets.

In reality, though, does it really matter if we achieve the sometimes impossible sounding targets suggested in the various guidelines? And are there any guidelines to help us to decide on how best to manage hypertension once it is diagnosed?

In answer to the first question, yes it does matter. The evidence from studies such as HOPE[1] and PROGRESS[2] shows that lower is better when it comes to blood pressure. The benefits of treatment can be seen in fewer cases of coronary heart disease (CHD) and cerebrovascular events (CVE). Lowering blood pressure in other diseases (renal disease, diabetes) also leads to better outcomes. Improving outcomes in diabetes means fewer long term complications such as blindness, amputations and dialysis or renal transplants. It is important to remember that the targets needed to achieve QOF points for the GMS contract are audit standards, i.e. they are the minimum acceptable levels of control that should be aimed for. The contract does state explicitly, however, that tighter control should be aimed for where possible.

As for the issue of which treatment guideline to use, the latest guidelines from NICE have been developed alongside the British Hypertension Society (BHS), so it would seem reasonable to use these guidelines as the standard. These guidelines can be accessed via the British Hypertension Society website at **www.bhsoc.org/Latest_BHS_management_Guidelines.stm**

Case study 4: Cheryl

Cheryl is a 51 year old lady who works as a practice nurse. She attends for a Well Woman check, as she has recently put on weight. She is, however, motivated to change. During this consultation you note that her blood pressure is 158/96.

In order to be certain that this is a reliable reading, care must be taken with making the measurement itself. Many factors can affect the reliability of this reading, and these factors may relate to both Cheryl herself and the machine that is used. Too many people are incorrectly diagnosed and managed because of poor blood pressure measurement technique.

Technique advice for measuring blood pressure with both mercury and digital sphygmomanometers from the British Hypertension Society can be found on the British Hypertension Society website.

Cheryl needs a full assessment of her health, lifestyle and risk factors. This might include bloods, ECG and repeated readings over the next month to rule out white coat hypertension. White coat hypertension may carry its own risks, however, and should not be dismissed as being unimportant.

Cheryl could be offered a home monitor to measure her readings away from the surgery or could be attached to an ambulatory blood pressure monitor which would measure her readings over a 24 hour period. The general advice, included in both the BHS/NICE guidelines and the Joint British Society Guidelines (JBS2), for interpreting home BP readings is that approximately

10mm/Hg should be added to the systolic figure and 5mm/Hg added to the diastolic figure before interpreting the significance of home readings. This reflects the fact that studies on the significance of raised BP readings are usually measured in a clinical setting; we therefore need to 'correct' for home readings, which will normally be lower than readings in the surgery. Another important pointer to look for is a night-time dip in 24 hour readings. It is part of normal physiology that we get a night-time dip of 10% in our blood pressure; the absence of this dip has been shown to correlate with increased morbidity and will identify those most likely to benefit from treatment.

Cheryl's blood results were essentially normal apart from a slight increase in her liver function test results, including her gamma GT. After gentle questioning Cheryl admitted that she had been drinking a bottle of wine on most nights as her husband worked away a lot. Her blood pressure remained borderline at around 146/90 but her ambulatory monitor showed a preserved nocturnal dip. She decided to try hard to cut down on her alcohol intake, once she realised that it was the likely cause of her raised BP. She also decided to follow the DASH diet (Dietary Approaches to Stop Hypertension) to improve her general health and reduce her blood pressure. As a result, her liver function tests returned to normal, her weight came down and her last BP reading was 142/86. Cheryl will benefit from regular monitoring in the future as a reading of 140/90 or more is generally considered to be outside of the ideal range.

Case study 5: Dora

Dora is a 78 year old lady who has hypertension. She is currently treated with bendroflumethiazide 5mg and atenolol 100mg, a combination which she has taken for over 10 years now. She rarely attends surgery as she doesn't like to be a bother but she has come to see the healthcare assistant (HCA) for a blood pressure check after getting a letter from you. The HCA is concerned to see that her BP reading is 169/102. Other medication includes: salbutamol inhaler - two puffs prn, Co-codamol effervescent - two tablets qds prn, and lactulose - 20ml bd.

It is important to be certain that the BP has been measured correctly using the appropriate size cuff and that three readings have been taken, spaced a minute apart, with the first one discarded before taking an average of the second and third readings. Once you have ensured that this is the case, you need to consider Dora's pharmacological and non-pharmacological management. In this case there are several areas for concern in her drug treatment.

The combination of thiazide diuretic and atenolol has been linked to higher levels of diabetes in the ASCOT[3] study so should be discouraged. Bendroflumethiazide should not normally be used in doses higher than 2.5mg, as doses above this have been linked to increased side effects with no additional benefit in terms of BP control. Furthermore, the use of a beta blocker and a B2 agonist (salbutamol) is questionable. When did the B2 agonist use start? Did Dora develop a tight chest or wheeze after starting on her beta blocker? This is a well known side effect and would suggest that the beta blocker should be stopped. The use of combination analgesia is generally discouraged (see **www.bnf.org.uk** for details). The codeine in co-codamol may not be useful or necessary, and may also be leading to the constipation for which Dora takes lactulose.

Finally, and very importantly, the 'fizz' that comes from the effervescent tablets is due to the inclusion of sodium in the formulation – more than 14mmol per tablet. If Dora takes eight tablets a day she will have exceeded the adult daily recommended sodium intake (100mmol) before she eats or drinks anything else. Stopping the co-codamol will reduce her salt intake, which in itself may reduce her blood pressure. By altering her therapy in this simple way you could:

- ◆ Reduce the number of drugs being taken and thus improve concordance
- ◆ Reduce the BP by reducing salt intake and thus reduce the number of anti-hypertensives needed
- ◆ Reduce the potential side effects of the drugs and thus improve concordance
- ◆ Reduce the risk of Dora going on to suffer a cardiovascular event
- ◆ Reduce the cost of therapy to the NHS

The final number of drugs that Dora could end up on could be just two – bendroflumethiazide 2.5mg and paracetamol. In reality, however, many people will need two or three anti-hypertensive drugs in order to reach the optimum BP target. This is perfectly acceptable and should not be seen as a failure. Indeed, it could be argued that patients should be warned about the likelihood of needing more than one tablet right from the time they are diagnosed with hypertension.

Case study 6: Otis

Otis is a 54 year old Afro-Caribbean man. He attended surgery for a wound dressing and an opportunistic BP check has shown that his BP is 179/96. He was reviewed a week later and his BP was 172/100. He failed to attend for his next appointment a week later but did appear the week after that when his BP was 166/97. He has no obvious lifestyle risk factors which need amending but you are aware that the traditional Afro Caribbean diet has been shown to have a high salt content, so you advise him about this. You are also aware that the Afro Caribbean population have a high incidence of hypertension, diabetes and stroke and together you decide that it is important to start on treatment. Which drug will you choose?

Treatment should be based around the NICE/BHS algorithm. Using this algorithm, a calcium channel blocker or a diuretic would be first choice for Otis as he is black. Common choices might include felodipine or amlodipine. If Otis cannot tolerate these drugs (common side effects include ankle oedema and flushing) he could try lercanidipine, which has fewer side effects and may be better tolerated. If a diuretic is chosen then it would usually be a thiazide diuretic such as bendroflumethiazide, which is cheap and effective but may impact on his lifestyle if an increased diuresis occurs and may have other side effects such as gout, erectile dysfunction and renal impairment – these are all relatively rare, however. If the BP is inadequately controlled on this therapy the next move would be to add an ACE inhibitor (or an angiotensin receptor blocker if the ACE inhibitor causes cough). Step three would be to add the remaining drug of the three which has not already been added so that you end up with an A + C + D combination - ACE plus Calcium channel blocker plus Diuretic. A new class of treatment for hypertension has recently been added to the armoury of drugs for hypertension: aliskiren, a renin inhibitor, works on the renin-angiotensin-aldosterone system (RAAS) and has been endorsed by the BHS for use in the management of hypertension.

If control remains elusive, however, it would be wise to consider referral for further advice. Most people with hypertension have so-called 'essential hypertension', where there is no known cause. However, in cases where the condition is particularly difficult to treat, in spite of optimal doses of medication and a multi-drug approach to getting readings down, it is important to consider the possibility of an underlying cause. Secondary hypertension is only seen in about 5% of all cases. Possible causes may include:

◆ Renal and reno-vascular disease

◆ Cushing's syndrome

◆ Conn's syndrome

◆ Phaechromocytoma

If blood pressure cannot be controlled with three different drug therapies then referral to a specialist should be seriously considered before adding in a 4th treatment group. This will allow further investigation of possible causes, such as those mentioned above.

Other possible causes include some types of medication being taken by the patient and it can be useful to check to see if any of these drugs are being used, as some are available over the counter and others may have been prescribed elsewhere.

Common drugs which can cause or exacerbate hypertension include:

◆ Oral steroids

◆ The oral contraceptive pill

- Decongestants such as pseudoephidrine
- Non-steroidal anti-inflammatory drugs

Interestingly, cocaine can cause acute hypertension, although it has not been linked to chronic hypertension.

Combination therapies are not used often in the UK, which is a shame when you consider the benefits to the patient of taking one tablet instead of two. Various arguments are given for this but it is interesting to note that whilst the search continues for the Holy Grail that is the diabetes 'Polypill', containing four or more ingredients, we largely ignore the potential benefits of combination therapy in hypertension management.

The issue of concordance is important when trying to work out why people do not reach target BP readings. It is vital to remember that behind all of these blood pressure readings and treatment is a person. People who have to take anti-hypertensive therapy are almost always on treatment for life for a condition which was not actually giving them any symptoms. This is difficult enough, but when that treatment itself gives side effects (as some of them may do) it must be even more difficult to 'keep taking the tablets'. One of the commonest reasons why people fail to reach blood pressure targets is a simple failure to take the treatment. This may be intentional or unintentional.

Intentional non-compliance includes deciding not to take a thiazide diuretic when travelling to avoid the nuisance factor of having to pass water more frequently on the journey. Unintentional non-compliance includes forgetting to take the drugs or failing to understand that the treatment is life-long rather than a 'course' and that treatment must continue, even if blood pressure reaches target levels.

In summary, then, it can be notoriously difficult to reach the targets suggested for optimal BP control but there is strong evidence to encourage us to do this. The best chance of reaching target comes from a 'joined-up' approach, which involves patients and professionals, lifestyle changes and optimisation of therapy; this includes accepting that polypharmacy may be a necessary price to pay for better BP control and lower rates of cardiovascular disease, and the many other complications of poorly controlled hypertension.

References

1. The Heart Outcomes Prevention Study Investigators *NEJM* 2000; 342: 145-153

2. PROGRESS Collaborative Group *Lancet* 2001; 358: 1033-1041

3. ASCOT (The Anglo-Scandinavian cardiac outcomes trial) *Lancet* 2005; 366: 895-906

Further reading

Hands on Hypertension: Getting to Targets in Practice *BJPCN* Volume 4, Number 5, September-October 2007

The ABC of Hypertension (2007), Beevers G, Lip G, O'Brien E. Blackwell Publishing

The DASH diet for hypertension (2003) (useful for patients, as well as health professionals) Moore T *et al.* Pocket Books Publishing

Further information

For more information on all aspects of hypertension go to the British Hypertension Society website at: *www.bhsoc.org*

To view the NICE/BHS guidelines go to: *www.nice.org.uk*

To access the JBS2 guidelines go to: *www.bcs.com/download/651/JBS2final.pdf*

For more information on the salt content of medicines go to: *www.nelm.nhs.uk/Documents/QA145.1%20-%20Sodiumcontent.doc?id=573370*

Chapter 4

Erectile dysfunction as a predictor of CVD

Patient presenting with ED but no current evidence of CVD; case study will focus on the link between the two, conditions and the role of risk assessment, and risk factor management to reduce risk.

Case study 7: Bob

Bob, 58, came in asking for an 'MOT' as he felt that he was at that age where 'everything starts to go wrong'. On further questioning, he reveals that his relationship is under pressure as he is unable to maintain an erection for long enough to complete an episode of intercourse. His wife thinks he has gone off her and suspects him of having an affair.

Erectile dysfunction (ED) occurs when a man is unable to maintain an erection which is adequate for penetration and/or successful intercourse. It is a relatively common condition and many men will experience an episode of ED at some time in their lives. Recurrent episodes can have a significant effect on quality of life, however, and treatment should therefore be considered for every man who seeks help.

However, there is another important issue connected to the subject of ED and that is the associated risk of cardiovascular disease. The penis has been called the barometer of cardiovascular health, as the vessels within the penis can be affected by cardio-vascular disease (CVD) in the same way as the heart (coronary heart disease), the brain (cerebrovascular disease) and the legs (peripheral arterial disease).

Recent research by Hodges et al (2007) has identified the fact that ED precedes CVD events by five years on average. This gives us a five-year window to reduce cardiovascular events, simply by identifying those men who have a history of ED. Vascular disease has also been identified as a leading cause of ED (Billups, 2005), so treatment of CVD risk factors should reduce both the risk of ED and the risk of a cardiovascular event. The risk factors themselves should be the same: age, smoking history, hypertension, dyslipidaemia, abnormal glycaemic control, and central obesity.

In the study by Hodges et al, 66% of men attending CVD rehabilitation groups reported an average of around five years' of symptomatic ED prior to their cardiovascular event, whereas 37% of an age-matched control group suffered from ED. In both groups, about half had actually discussed their ED with a health professional. Sadly, in those men who went on to suffer a cardiovascular event, the ED got worse.

This indicates that we need to identify ED in otherwise asymptomatic men who are at risk of a future cardiovascular event and that we then need uncompromising and aggressive treatment of their risk factors as suggested by the JBS2 publication for people at high risk. Careful history taking and identification of those men who suffer from ED is vital as they often fail to discuss it with their healthcare professional. It is crucial, then, that we seek out information about ED in order to treat both the condition itself and the associated cardiovascular risk effectively.

Broaching the subject of ED

The fact that many men with ED do not discuss their problem with their healthcare professional means that we should make a habit of routinely and proactively introducing the subject into a range of consultations. However, one of the commonest concerns for health professionals dealing with ED is broaching the subject. Nurses often say that they feel that the issue is taboo. It can be especially difficult for some nurses to discuss the subject with older men, as people still feel that sex in the elderly population is a sensitive subject. It can be easier to open discussions around ED when you are already in the person's 'personal space', for instance when taking observations such as BP and pulse or when undertaking waist measurements. Another method for introducing the subject is to say 'Some men who smoke/have high blood pressure/have raised cholesterol have problems with getting and keeping an erection; is that a problem for you?' This will highlight those individuals who have ED and are at risk of CVD but who are unable or unwilling to mention this to members of the healthcare team.

In the Global Study of Sexual Attitudes and Behaviours **(GSSAB)** study in 2002, the prevalence of occasional, periodic or frequent ED in men age 40-80 years of age was 17.5%, with an increased prevalence as the men got older. The same study confirmed that significant numbers of men and women still remained interested in having an active sex life into their 80s. However, before starting treatment for ED it is important to ascertain whether the couple actually want treatment for the problem. Up to one in five men and one in three women do not actually want a sexual relationship. Added difficulties come when one partner wants treatment but the other does not wish to re-engage in a sexual relationship. This requires very sensitive handling, and referral to a relationship counsellor may be useful.

Treating ED

Treatment options for ED will depend on the likely cause, and fall into two main categories:

- Pharmacological, including tablets, intercavernosal injections and urethral pellets

- Non-pharmacological, including splints, pumps, vibrators and psychosexual relationship counselling

Pharmacological therapies

There are two main drug classes used to treat ED; the first is the Phosphodiesterase 5 (PDE5) inhibitors, which include sildenafil (Viagra), tadalafil (Cialis) and vardenafil (Levitra); the second is the Prostaglandin E1 therapy, alprostadil.

PDE5 inhibitors are the first line recommended treatment for ED. Sildenafil works by relaxing smooth muscle in the corpus cavernosal, thus allowing blood to flow into the penis. Sexual stimulation is necessary to get the drug to work – it will not work alone. It is available in 25mcg, 50mcg and 100mcg doses and takes effect within 20-30 minutes, with peak effect at 60 minutes, so should be taken about an hour before sex. The usual starting dose is 50mg. It lasts for 4-6 hours and should only be used once daily. Side effects are often related to the vasodilatory action of the drug and include headache, dizziness and flushing. Other side effects include palpitations and visual disturbances. Recently, a very important but rare potential side effect of sildenafil has been recorded. This is known as non-arteritic ischaemic optic atrophy and can lead to blindness. Men who are prescribed sildenafil should therefore be advised to report visual disturbances immediately.

Sildenafil interacts with nitrate-containing drugs, such as those prescribed in cardiovascular disease and including glycerine trinitrate (GTN) spray. If these drugs are given together, they can lead to a catastrophic drop in blood pressure which can be fatal. Sildenafil, along with the other PDE5 inhibitors, should not be taken with food or grapefruit juice.

Tadalafil works in the same way as sildenafil but onset of action occurs after about 60 minutes, with a peak effect at two hours after taking it. It lasts 12-48 hours. In other respects the action of the drug and the possible side effects are similar to sildenafil, although there have been some reports of muscle aches and back pain with tadalafil. It should also not be used with clarithromycin. It is available in doses of 10mg and 20mg; the usual starting dose is 10mg taken 1-2 hours before sex, although timing is less important due to its length of action.

Vardenafil is available in doses of 5mg, 10mg and 20mg with the effect lasting between 4-6 hours. The usual dose is 10mg 30-60 minutes before sex.

The PDE5 inhibitors should not be taken with food as this can inhibit their action. The manufacturers of Cialis claim that this is less evident with their drug. The decision about which dose to use will depend on the individual presentation of the patient, but if the initial dose does not work then the next dose up should be tried, after checking with the patient that the drug was used correctly. Some patients forget that stimulation is part of the requirement of ensuring that the drug works.

The second class of drug used to treat ED is the prostaglandin E1, a naturally occurring substance needed for a healthy erection, which is given in the form of alprostadil. Alprostadil may be delivered via an injection into the shaft of the penis (Caverject or Viridal) or a pellet inserted into the urethra (MUSE). In both cases, the user must be taught correct administration techniques by a trained professional prior to self-administration.

Caverject (alprostadil 5mcg, 10mcg, 20mcg) or Viridal (alprostadil 10, 20 or 40mcg) is injected directly into the body of the penis but is surprisingly well tolerated by those men who try it – they often find that it is almost painless. An erection will usually follow within 15 minutes, which will last approximately an hour. It is successful in 90% of men who try it but it will not suit all men, mainly because of the method itself. For men who want to try it but are squeamish about injecting themselves, their partner can be taught the technique if they are willing to learn. The injection can be used up to three times a week maximum, leaving at least 24 hours between uses.

MUSE stands for Medicated Urethral System for Erection and consists of small pellets inserted into the urethral opening, ideally after passing urine, as this affords a little lubrication. The pellets contain alprostadil 125mcg, 250mcg, 500mcg and 1000mg, of which 250mcg is the usual starting dose. They work in 5-20 minutes and last up to an hour. Success rates and acceptability vary in the men who try them. They can be used up to twice daily but must be spaced out and are not suitable to be used consecutively without a break. No more than seven treatments should be used in one week.

Alprostadil can cause penile discomfort and prolonged erections in some men.

Non-pharmacological approaches

These include splints, vacuum pumps and rings, vibrators and relationship therapy. Of these the choice of intervention will depend on the user. Vacuum pumps can be used to draw blood into the penis and the ring is then used to trap the blood in. Vibrators can induce erection and orgasm, even in people with spinal injuries. Splinting involves insertion of a splint under anaesthetic but can also lead to destruction of the erectile tissue. Psychosexual counselling is more likely to be effective in people with anxiety and depression-related ED than in those with underlying physiological disorders such as vascular disease.

Prescribing restrictions for ED

The British National Formulary **(www.bnf.org)** states that none of these drugs are prescribable on the NHS, unless they are prescribed to treat erectile dysfunction in men who:

- have diabetes, multiple sclerosis, Parkinson's disease, poliomyelitis, prostate cancer, severe pelvic injury, single gene neurological disease, spina bifida, or spinal cord injury

- are receiving dialysis for renal failure

- have had radical pelvic surgery, prostatectomy (including transurethral resection of the prostate), or kidney transplant

- were receiving treatments for erectile dysfunction, at the expense of the NHS, on 14 September 1998

- are suffering severe distress as a result of impotence. Severe distress should be diagnosed in a specialist centre and is defined as that which causes significant disruption to normal social and occupational activities; a marked effect on mood, behaviour, social and environmental awareness, or a marked effect on interpersonal relationships.

There are several ways in which ED can be linked to cardiovascular disease. Firstly it can be, as demonstrated above, a direct result of atherosclerotic disease; secondly, it can be linked to diabetes, which may in itself precede CVD. Thirdly, it can occur as the result of the use of drug treatments for CVD. So it may be relatively easy to ask someone who has diabetes if they have ED, as this is part of a routine diabetes management review. However, these people are already known to be at high risk of CVD and should therefore be receiving the full range of pharmacological and non-pharmacological interventions known to reduce cardiovascular risk. In the same way, men who take beta blockers and diuretics, amongst other drugs, should be advised about the possibility of drug induced ED and should be asked to report any symptoms.

The real challenge, though, comes from actively discussing ED with patients who do not fall into one of these groups. The government is focusing on risk assessment for the population, using risk assessment tables such as JBS2 or websites such as **www.qrisk.org** so the profile of ED as another cardiovascular risk factor should be highlighted amongst the public and healthcare professionals alike. Cardiovascular disease is also a disease linked to deprivation and we know that people in deprived areas are less likely to eat healthily, take regular exercise, avoid smoking and maintain alcohol levels within safe limits, all of which will put them at increased risk of CVD. Another challenge, then, is to get risk assessment activities out into the community rather than expecting people to come to the health service provider for assessment and intervention. In Birmingham, a pilot study has been set up within community pharmacies to increase the numbers of people having their cardiovascular risk assessment done who would not normally access healthcare. The study has already shown that a significant number of people using this service are not even registered with a GP, so those in most need are those with least access to care.

Reducing risk

Reducing cardiovascular risk involves identifying potential triggers for CVD and treating them with medication and lifestyle changes to reduce that risk. Treating these factors can also impact on ED itself (Rosen et al, 2005). Known modifiable risk factors and appropriate interventions are listed below:

Table 4.1: Modifiable risk factors for CVD and appropriate interventions

Smoking

Drug treatment	Lifestyle advice	Other
NRT, buproprion, varenicline	Behavioural support to quit	Combination of both works best

Dyslipidaemia

Statin, ezetimibe, fibrate, nicotinic acid, resin	Healthy diet, low saturated fat, exercise to increase HDL	Reduce total cholesterol to <5 (< 4 if possible) and LDL to <3 (<2 if possible)

Hypertension

As per British hypertension/NICE guidelines	Healthy diet, exercise, care with alcohol and salt intake	2 or 3 drugs often needed to reach BP targets

Central obesity

Orlistat or sibutramine if appropriate	Low saturated fat, reduced calorie diet	Behavioural support needed along with dietary and activity modification

Hyperglycaemia

Hypoglycaemic drug, e.g. metformin in diagnosed type 2 diabetes	Healthy, sugar free, low saturated fat diet with exercise to improve insulin sensitivity	

Alcohol

N/A	Keep within safe drinking limits	Advice on behavioural change available in NICE guidance 10/07

Activity levels

N/A	30 mins five times a week is ideal; this can be split into two shorter sessions, if preferred	A brisk walk with the family or the dog after school or work each day will do the job. 20 mins exercise improves insulin sensitivity for 15 hours afterwards

Self help

For those people who do not like to come into a surgery or clinic, there is an online risk assessment tool that can be used to estimate cardiovascular risk and show the potential improvement that can be gained from a range of interventions. Qrisk (www.qrisk.org) can be used by anyone to assess individual risk using known risk factors such as hypertension, lipid levels, age, sex, smoking and family history. Whatever the initial score, people will be advised how to reduce their risk and may then be encouraged to make lifestyle changes or to access healthcare services for further advice and intervention.

References

Billups KL (2005) Sexual Dysfunction and Cardiovascular Disease: Integrative Concepts and Strategies. *The American Journal of Cardiology* Volume 96, Issue 12, Supplement 2, p57-61

Hodges, L.D. et al (2007) The temporal relationship between erectile dysfunction and cardiovascular disease. *International Journal of Clinical Practice*; 61: 12, 2019-2025

Rosen RC, Friedman M and Kostis JB (2005) Lifestyle Management of Erectile Dysfunction: The Role of Cardiovascular and Concomitant Risk Factors. *The American Journal of Cardiology* Volume 96, Issue 12, Supplement 2, p76-79

Further information

British hypertension society/NICE guidelines available from: *www.nice.org.uk* and from: *www.bhsoc.org*

Advice re lipids can be found at: *www.heartuk.org.uk*

Joint British Society Guidelines 2 (JBS2) available from: *www.heartjnl.com*

A British Heart Foundation factfile on JBS2 can be found at: *www.bhsoc.org/bhf_factfiles/bhf_factfile_jan_2006.pdf*

Case study 8: Mike

Mike is a 48 year old Afro Caribbean man who is married with a three year old son. He has a long history of asthma, which has been well controlled on a combination of an inhaled steroid and a long acting b2 agonist. Mike normally attends for his annual asthma review and in between times if he feels that his asthma is less well controlled. He arrives in surgery on this occasion complaining of increased shortness of breath, particularly at night. He claims that he is taking his inhaler as normal and that he cannot think of any reason why his asthma has suddenly got worse.

Things you might need to consider now include:

- Review of inhaler technique

- Compliance/concordance issues

- Exposure to new irritants: decorating or building materials within the home; change of job with occupational irritants; new pets; season change; poorly controlled allergic rhinitis

- Current peak flow readings versus best peak flow reading and/or peak flow diary

- Existence of other symptoms to strengthen or contradict the likelihood of asthma being the cause of his breathlessness

Mike tells you he has been taking his blue reliever inhaler more than four times a day and that he has increased the dose of his combination treatment for the past week on the instructions of one of the GPs in the practice last week. He still feels no better. Surprisingly, however, his peak flow remains within 90% of his best ever reading.

What could you do next?

- You could take a further history

- You could undertake a physical examination

- You could request some investigations

Let's look at the possible benefits of taking each of these approaches:

Further history

It's important to get a thorough history from Mike. This would include the history of the presenting complaint, any past medical history and any drug history, including prescribed therapy, over the counter treatments and complementary therapies, and finally any recreational drug use, including social drugs such as cigarettes and alcohol. Information about his family history can be useful and psycho-social history might prove useful too. Mike said that he only drinks occasionally (less than once a week) and when he does it is only 1-2 units a day. He used to smoke heavily but has stopped since his 30th birthday. He takes no medication other than his inhalers, and he has no significant past medical history. There is a family history of type 2 diabetes and stroke on his mother's side.

Physical examination

It has been said that history is 80% of your diagnosis but a thorough physical examination of the patient can help to confirm or refute a possible diagnosis through the presence or absence of certain physical signs. In Mike's case he was seen to be suffering from some shortness of breath, reportedly worse at night. He was also very overweight with a body mass index of 36 and a waist circumference of 112cm. Because of this, further examination of the chest and abdomen proved both difficult and inconclusive, although there were inspiratory crackles in the chest. Jugular venous pressure was increased to 5cm and there was evidence of ankle oedema. A third heart sound was listened for but not detected. Observations included a temperature of 37.1, pulse of 108 with a regular rhythm, respiratory rate of 32 and blood pressure of 173/99 which persisted after three readings.

Tests and investigations

These might initially include:

+ An ECG in view of the dyspnoea, inspiratory crackles and ankle oedema. All of these symptoms are suggestive of possible heart failure

+ Lung function tests such as peak expiratory flow readings and spirometry

+ Blood tests to include full blood count, kidney and liver function, blood glucose, lipids, ESR/CKP/CRP variants

+ Chest X-ray

+ Blood gases via pulse oximetry or referral arterial blood gases

Of course, a combination of these approaches affords the best chance of getting the diagnosis correct and therefore ensuring optimum treatment and management of the condition.

Mike was referred to the heart failure clinic after his ECG showed left ventricular hypertrophy. He was diagnosed with heart failure after his echocardiogram showed an ejection fraction of 35%. After optimisation of his drug treatment, using maximum doses of ACE inhibitors, diuretics for fluid control and a trial of very low dose beta blockers, which was unsuccessful due to his asthma, the decision was made that he would benefit from insertion of an implantable device. Mike was admitted for assessment of his suitability for a biventricular pacemaker and defibrillator.

Dying for your help: the psychological impact of heart failure

Living with a long term condition (LTC) is the reality for thousands of people in the UK. As the population ages and more people survive events which might have been fatal in the past, this number is likely to continue to rise. Much has been written about what needs to be done about this, but the focus is often on the importance of reducing admissions and managing LTCs better in the community. Whilst this aim is laudable it assumes that much of the morbidity of LTCs is treatable and avoidable. In heart failure, for example, there is much discussion about the role of optimising drug therapies to improve outcomes and reduce acute admissions resulting from decompensated heart failure. A lot of this management centres on the person with heart failure being involved in self managing their condition with daily weights, drug titration, fluid restriction and careful attention to diet and activity levels. What do you do, then, when the person you're trying to engage in active self-management turns around to you and says: 'Actually, love, I'm alright. Just leave me alone. It's my time and I'm ready to die.'

Case study 9: Alex

Alex is 88 years old and was married for 63 years before his wife died five years ago. He now lives alone with his budgie, although he has occasional visits from his daughter and granddaughter. He was diagnosed with heart failure after a bout of pneumonia last year. He is currently taking furosemide 40mg in the morning, ramipril 10mg and nebivolol 5mg. The furosemide makes him 'pee for England' as he puts it and he complains of feeling very tired at times – he puts this down to sleeping badly. He lives on food which he orders from a 'Meals on Wheels' type private supplier. He enjoys a cigarette and a whisky at night to help him relax.

You are concerned that Alex is sleeping badly because of orthopnoea and you want to increase the dose of furosemide but Alex is adamant that he does not want any further intervention. You suspect that he may in fact be depressed.

What can you do?

The first thing to do is to perform a formal assessment of Alex's psychological status to see whether or not he is actually depressed. There are a few accredited tools which can be used to do this, such as the Hospital Anxiety and Depression Scale (HADS) or the PHQ9 tool. Using a tool to assess for depression is important as it will help identify clinical depression as opposed to the general and, one could argue, normal feelings of sadness that might accompany Alex's diagnosis.

So why does it matter if Alex is depressed? This subject was covered in some depth at a recent American Cardiology Society conference. Studies presented at the conference described how the presence of depression in people with heart failure leads to worse outcomes and even death. The GMS contract awards points for assessing for depressive illness in patients with diabetes or coronary heart disease. However, it seems that even in the absence of a points value, it would be worth assessing people with heart failure for depression too. Various studies estimate that anywhere from 24-42% of heart failure patients also suffer from depression.

In those people with a pre-existing diagnosis of depression the risks are even higher and the importance of controlling the depression, as well as the heart failure symptoms, must be stressed. It is also vital to remember that many people with heart failure will be housebound or may live in sheltered accommodation or nursing homes, and these people may be at greater risk of slipping through the net. Patients with both heart failure and depression are at higher risk of suffering or dying from a transient ischaemic attack, stroke or heart attack and are at greater risk of requiring re-admission than those who have heart failure alone.

Why does depression increase risk?

It is unclear why this should be. Some studies suggest that there may be pathophysiological reasons that lead to an increased tendency to clot or to develop arrhythmias. Others suggest that the reasons are related to behavioural issues, including a reduced concordance rate with treatments and lifestyle measures aimed at improving symptoms and outcomes. A recent study[1] from the American Heart Journal showed that the presence of depression in people with heart disease can lead to higher levels of certain inflammatory protein markers, which may then increase their risk of dying.

The protein, known as tumour necrosis factor alpha (TNF-a), belongs to the family known as cytokines and there has long been a suspicion that raised levels of cytokines are related to an increased risk of depression. This new study goes further and suggests that high levels of TFN-a may indicate those people who are at higher risk of dying, as the inflammation caused by TFN-a may further impair the heart's ability to pump effectively. In a study of 32 people with heart failure, the 14 patients who felt the most depressed had almost twice the levels of TFN-a in their blood. Thirty-two patients from the heart failure clinic at Ohio State were recruited and answered the 21-question Beck Depression Inventory, another tool used to measure symptoms of depression. Answers to each question are given a value of nil (no symptoms at all) to 3 (severe symptoms). A score of 10 or more suggests that a patient has at least mild symptoms of depression. Although the link between heart failure and depression is clear, what we don't know is whether depression causes the inflammation which leads to heart failure or if heart failure causes depression, which accelerates inflammation.

So what can we do with depressed heart failure patients?

There is limited evidence that interventions aimed at improving levels of depression in patients with heart failure leads to improved outcomes, although the general advice given is to treat using selective serotonin reuptake inhibitors (SSRIs) such as fluoxetine. Tricyclic antidepressants (TCAs) such as amitriptyline are usually avoided due to their cardiotoxic side effects along with other side effects such as a dry mouth, which can be particularly unpleasant in someone taking diuretics and who may also be on fluid restriction. It is important to recognise, though, that offering drug therapy for depression will mean the person with heart failure having to take yet another pill on top of the many tablets already being taken for the heart failure itself. The impact of yet another tablet should not be underestimated, especially as the depression itself will reduce the chance of good adherence to drug regimes and increase the risk of drug interactions.

The National Institute for Health and Clinical Excellence (NICE) state that an SSRI and/or cognitive behavioural therapy (CBT) should be the first line approach for treating depression. However, it is quite difficult to access CBT in many areas of the country, especially if the service user is housebound. Furthermore, there are no randomised controlled trails (RCTs) looking at the benefits of psychological interventions in heart failure. That does not mean that these interventions would not work, it simply means that no-one has looked into whether they work or not.

Improving Alex's social interactions may also help with his depression. Since the death of his wife and his diagnosis of pneumonia and heart failure he has limited opportunities to get out of the house. Some areas of the country encourage people with heart failure to attend cardiac rehabilitation courses, which can provide an excellent opportunity for meeting other people. Otherwise social services can often provide information about clubs and events that Alex may be able attend with help.

How might Alex's depression affect his heart failure?

With the accent on self management for people with long term conditions there is one important proviso in heart failure, but possibly in other conditions, such as Chronic Obstructive Pulmonary Disease (COPD). Most people with heart failure are elderly. The damaged pump will reduce the amount of blood getting around the body and this will include the cerebral circulation. A combination of ageing and impaired oxygenation of the cerebral tissues may well result in reduced cognitive abilities. It may be unfeasible, therefore, to expect all people with heart failure to self manage when this requires careful monitoring of body weight, fluid intake, symptoms and dose titration of diuretics. Self management is not always appropriate for all people and the fact that people may be unable to self manage and self medicate needs to be recognised as a potential cause of acute hospital admissions. Most hospital admissions for decompensated heart failure result from inadequate drug management, but it may not always be easy to avoid this.

In conclusion, then, depression is very common in people with heart failure, although it is often under-diagnosed. Alex has heart failure and may also have depression. Although there are no QOF points for assessing people with heart failure for depression, it is still important to do so as the presence of depression can double the risk of dying. It is important to make this assessment using an accredited tool; this will differentiate it from the 'normal' feelings of sadness which may accompany the diagnosis of a life threatening condition such as heart failure. If depression is diagnosed it is important to realise the significant impact this may have on Alex's outcome, and treatment should be offered. SSRIs can safely be used to treat depression in people who have heart failure.

Psychological approaches such as CBT can also be tried, although there is no evidence for their usefulness in improving heart failure outcomes. However, NICE recognises the value of CBT in depression generally. Overall, Alex's management should include an assessment of his mental health and his physical health. It should be recognised that cognitive impairment, with or without depression, may impact negatively on a person's ability to recognise the symptoms of heart failure and to self manage accordingly.

Reference

1. A.Ferketich, J.Ferguson, P.Binkley *American Heart Journal*, Volume 150, Issue 1, Pages 132-136

Case study 10: George

George is a 62 year old retired hospital porter who has a history of type 2 diabetes and hypertension. He takes metformin 500mg bd and ramipril 5mg. His blood pressure is not well controlled and his most recent reading was 154/93.

George attended surgery four months ago complaining of pins and needles and weakness in his arm following a game of squash. He mentioned that during this game he had played very badly as his vision had become blurred. His squash partner drove him home and he went to bed two hours later, as he was still having the symptoms, along with a headache. By the next morning he was better and attended the surgery for a check-up. He was diagnosed as having migraine and was advised accordingly. He has not been seen in the surgery since then.

He was, however, discharged from the stroke unit four weeks ago, having suffered a stroke which left him with a mild right hemiparesis and some residual expressive dysphasia. It is now thought that George's 'migraine' was actually a transient ischaemic attack – a 'mini-stroke' which can be the harbinger of a full blown stroke if left undiagnosed and untreated.

What else could have been done?

It is possible to use tools such as the ABCD scoring system to predict possible stroke after a TIA.

Table 6.1: ABCD scoring system to predict possible stroke after TIA

Age	Question	Score
A	<60 years	0
	≥60 years	1

Blood pressure	Question	Score
B	Systolic >140 mmHg and/or d diastolic ≥90 mmHg	1

Blinical features	Question	Score
C	Unilateral weakness	2
	Speech disturbance without weakness	1
	Other	0

Duration of symptoms	Question	Score
D	≥60 minutes	2
	10-59 minutes	1
	<10 minutes	0

Results of scoring

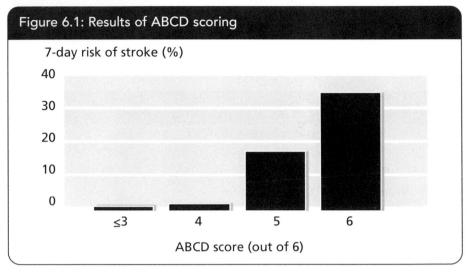

Figure 6.1: Results of ABCD scoring

7-day risk of stroke (%)

ABCD score (out of 6)

(From Bandolier: www.jr2.ox.ac.uk/bandolier/band139/b139-5.html)

Based on this system, George would have scored 6 points.

What do you need to know?

Understanding what has happened to George is vital. The hospital discharge summary states that George has suffered an ischaemic stroke, caused by a thrombus or embolus blocking the blood supply to the brain tissues. The type of stroke will dictate the type of treatment regime that should be offered.

How do we manage this condition in the long term?

From now on the aims of George's care will be to reduce the risk of further cardiovascular events and to minimise the impact of the stroke that George has already had. Patricia, the practice nurse, takes the time to review George's medication and discusses any concordance issues. George explained that he had not always been careful to take his medication as prescribed. He hated having to take tablets when 'he wasn't ill'. His stroke had reminded him of the reason for taking them and he was now determined to take them as prescribed. Patricia spent some time going through the tablets he was now taking and made sure that George and Claire, his wife, understood how and why he should take it. George was on a suboptimal dose of ramipril, both in terms of managing his hypertension and in terms of optimising cardiovascular protection. Patricia arranged for the dose to be uptitrated to 10mg and for subsequent blood pressure measurements and renal function to be checked.

Secondary prevention approaches need to be in place for all stroke patients unless contraindicated. These include lifestyle measures such as stopping smoking, keeping as active as possible and eating healthily. Patricia discussed these areas with George and Claire and made sure that they understood the importance of committing to a healthy lifestyle. Claire did most of the cooking and was aware of how to make healthy food choices, including fish, fruit and vegetables and a low salt intake. George was continuing with his physiotherapy since his discharge from hospital, and Claire had taken him to the golf course to meet up with friends and have a short walk around the 5th tee, which was his favourite. He said he was keen to get back to his golf in the future and Patricia encouraged this.

Lipid lowering treatment is also important in stroke prevention but George was not taking a statin, despite the updated guidelines on the management of type 2 diabetes from NICE (**www.nice.org.uk**), which recommend that all patients with type 2 diabetes over the age of 40 are prescribed statins unless they are low risk. Patricia will need to monitor lipid levels and liver function tests in the future and watch for any side effects of these drugs.

Antiplatelet therapy is another cornerstone in the treatment and prevention of stroke. A combination of aspirin and modified release dipyridamole, if tolerated, is recommended for two years following a transient ischaemic attack or stroke. If aspirin is not tolerated then clopidogrel alone can be used as an alternative. Again, the NICE guidelines advise that aspirin is offered to all patients with type 2 diabetes over the age of 50, although the POPADAD study *(Belch et al 2008)* disputed its value.

Bearing in mind the medication George was taking, Patricia gently asked George and Claire whether they had resumed their sex life since the stroke, and how things were going in this department. People may find the idea of physical closeness frightening after a stroke and may be worried about causing further harm. Patricia reassured the couple that there was no reason for delaying a resumption of their sex life if both partners were comfortable with the idea. George then explained that he had been having some problems with erectile dysfunction for a year before the stroke and that they were actually happy with a non-sexual, albeit close, relationship at present. Patricia resolved to return to this issue later in the year, in case they felt that they needed further advice or support. A useful booklet can be downloaded from Chest, Heart and Stroke Scotland (CHSS) on:
www.chss.org.uk/pdf/publications/stroke/SS6_Sex_after_stroke.pdf

Rehabilitation began in the immediate post-stroke period while George was still in hospital. However, this is an ongoing process and needs to continue now George has been discharged. Physiotherapy exercises must be carried out regularly if they are to have the maximum effect, and the focus will often be on using both sides of the body in order to avoid defaulting to the unaffected side and leaving the affected side unused and unimproved. Occupational therapy will also have been initiated in hospital but further input may be needed at home in order to optimise George's ability to perform the activities of daily living. Occupational therapists often use handicraft tasks and board games to improve spatial and memory skills. George was very fond of jigsaws before his stroke and the therapist encouraged him to indulge this hobby. The physiotherapist and the occupational therapist can also help George with problems caused by the blurred vision he has had since the stroke. Further input can be given by opticians and ophthalmologists.

George has continued to have speech therapy, as his speech had been affected by the stroke. He found it very frustrating not being able to communicate effectively, which was due to a combination of expressive dysphasia – meaning that he was unable to find the words he wanted in order to be able to say what he meant – and dysarthria, which meant that facial weakness affected his ability to form the words accurately. Speech therapists, along with community dieticians, can also ensure that George is able to manage to eat an adequate dietary and fluid intake, which is important for his general well being.

Other healthcare professionals that may be involved in George's care will include the district nursing service, community matrons, diabetes specialist nurse and health visitor. All of these individuals will need to co-ordinate their care, and Patricia is well placed to help conduct this orchestra of assistance. George will also be able to access support from social services, the voluntary sector and stroke support groups.

It is important that support is made available for Claire and not just for George. The impact of the stroke ripples through the entire family, not just the patient himself. Up until George had his stroke he was active and was still earning through his part time job at the golf course. Claire also worked as a part time waitress at the local hotel. George has been unable to continue in his job and Claire has also had to give up hers in order to look after him. This will have an effect on their financial situation and they may need to look into the possibility of getting financial support and advice. Just as important, however, is the effect on their self-esteem and their view of themselves as independent contributors to the world around them. George had suffered from depression since his stroke and this is not uncommon. Early diagnosis of the depression using a validated tool (in this case, the HADS score while he was in hospital) and treatment using fluoxetine meant that George has the best opportunity of recovering from his depression. Furthermore, Patricia was able to refer him for some cognitive behavioural therapy from the practice counsellor, which he found particularly useful.

George had been told about the local Expert Patient Programme in hospital and Patricia was happy to give them more information about the service. Claire was also encouraged to attend these sessions; she is still very distressed by George's stroke. She had found him collapsed on the floor after she had been at work at the local hotel and had dialled 999. She felt useless at the time and wondered, as she saw him disappear off in the ambulance, whether she would see him again. She confessed to Patricia recently that watching him struggle since the stroke was just as hard as wondering if he would survive at the time. Claire loved her job and is suffering a double loss – both of her husband's independence and of her own.

Patricia's involvement in George's and Claire's care is vital. She knows the couple well and is able to relate to them both, having known them before and after the event. She is able to ensure George gets the evidence based treatment he needs to reduce the risk of further strokes.

References

Cox, Beverley. Stroke and TIA management, *British Journal of Primary Care Nursing – Cardiovascular Disease and Diabetes*, Volume 4, Issue 2 March-April 2007 Pages 67-73. *www.bjpcn-cardiovascular.com*

Cox, Beverley. Optimising your patients' recovery after stroke *British Journal of Primary Care Nursing – Cardiovascular Disease and Diabetes*, Volume 5, Issue 3 May-June 2008 Pages 137-139. *www.bjpcn-cardiovascular.com*

Belch J, MacCuish A, Campbell I et al 2008. Prevention of progression of arterial disease and diabetes (POPADAD) *BMJ* 337; a1840

Case study 11: Agnes

Agnes is an 80 year old lady with a history of hypertension, chronic obstructive pulmonary disease (COPD) and heart failure. A recent echocardiogram showed an ejection fraction of 38%. She is treated with perindopril 8mg but was unable to tolerate a beta-blocker. One afternoon her daughter, Carrie, calls to say that Agnes is feeling unwell, although her symptoms are unspecific. She says she feels 'tired and under the weather' but is also complaining of a mild degree of breathlessness. The GP asks Carrie to bring Agnes down to the surgery to attend the first contact clinic for an initial assessment.

What sort of examination and investigations might be useful?

Agnes needs a full assessment. This would include taking a history of the current complaint, as well as a record of past medical history. With Carrie's help, Agnes explains that she has been feeling out of sorts and out of puff for several days now but is unable to give any further example of specific symptoms. She smoked 20-30 a day between the ages of 18 and 64. She is not overweight and she drinks the occasional sherry on special occasions only. On examination her BP is unrecordable as the electronic machine keeps saying 'error'. The GP decides to use the mercury sphygmomanometer, as the digital machine is playing up, and realises, when she put her fingers on her wrist, that her pulse is 98 bpm and irregular. A quick glance at her records tells her that this irregular pulse has never been commented on before. Recognising that she may have an undiagnosed arrhythmia the GP arranges for Agnes to have an ECG.

Learning point

Digital sphygmomanometers will not record blood pressure accurately if the patient has an arrhythmia. It is important to recognise that if the machine is not recording the blood pressure and an 'error' message is received, then further investigations should be carried out to exclude an arrythmia such as atrial fibrillation. One of the problems with using digital machines is that it is easy to omit checking the pulse or to rely on the machine for a rate without checking the rhythm.

Diagnosis

The NICE guidelines state that all patients with an irregular pulse should have an ECG as a means of detecting AF. Stacey, the healthcare assistant, records an ECG. The strip looks like this:

Figure 7.1: ECG Strip

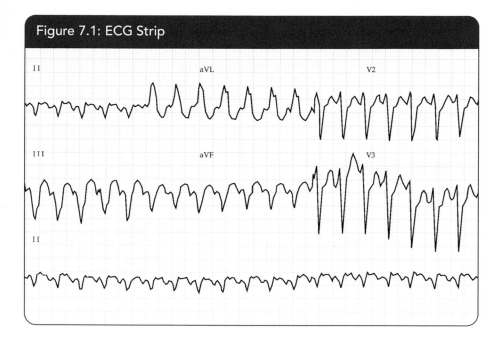

The GP realises that the ECG shows a rapid, irregular, narrow QRS complex tachycardia with absent P waves which is diagnostic of atrial fibrillation. Bearing in mind the importance of ECGs in diagnosing AF, a recent study showed that some GPs and nurses have difficulty diagnosing AF on ECG, leading to inappropriate treatment for patients.

The SAFE study (Hobbs et al, 2005) asked 50 GPs and nurses to assess the presence of AF in a set of ECGs randomly selected from a pool of 1,696. The diagnoses were then confirmed by cardiologists. GPs performed better than nurses, possibly because of greater experience in this area. They correctly diagnosed 79 of 99 cases of atrial fibrillation but also incorrectly diagnosed 114 ECGs as showing AF when they showed sinus rhythm, giving a positive predictive value of just 41%. There may be an argument, then, for the need for further training for GPs and nurses, or alternatively for allowing easier access to specialists who have accredited expertise in this area.

AF occurs when the atria of the heart beat in a chaotic, irregular and rapid way which leads to an irregular rhythm with a weakened force of contraction. This can result in a 10-25% reduction in cardiac output. AF is more common in men than women. Overall, the risk increases with age. Although the condition may be asymptomatic, a careful history may reveal signs and symptoms which may warrant further investigations. A manual pulse check can reveal an irregular pulse in those who are asymptomatic. Alternatively, patients may complain of a variety of symptoms during episodes of AF, and these may be fairly non-specific. They can include breathlessness, palpitations, dizziness, transient ischaemic attacks and chest pain.

AF may occur with no identifiable cause – this is known as lone AF. However, there are several known risk factors for the development of this common arrhythmia. These include:

- Hypertension, especially with left ventricular hypertrophy

- Heart failure, particularly within past three months

- Diabetes mellitus

- Previous history of transient ischaemic attack or stroke

- BMI of 30 or above

- Alcohol intake of 42 units or more per week

- Chronic respiratory disease

- Hyperthyroidism

(Ruigómez et al, 2002).

Agnes' risk factors include her age, gender, hypertension, COPD and heart failure.

What will you do next?

According to the NICE Atrial Fibrillation care pathway (**www.nice.org.uk**) Agnes needs further assessment, including blood tests, to include a full blood count, urea and electrolytes, liver function tests, thyroid function tests, glucose and lipid profile. These are done in order to exclude metabolic and thyroid disorders and electrolyte imbalance, all of which are more common in the elderly population and which may predispose Agnes to AF. Agnes's blood pressure, using the mercury sphygmomanometer, is 166/94 mm/Hg.

Other investigations may include:

◆ A coagulation screen to assess suitability for anticoagulation and as a baseline

◆ 24 hour ECG monitoring or an event recorder ECG if paroxysmal AF is suspected

◆ Chest X-ray to identify underlying lung disease or evidence of cardiomegaly, which may indicate the possible presence of heart failure

◆ Echocardiography to identify underlying abnormalities such as structural defects or left ventricular dysfunction, which may affect treatment choices

Agnes's results reveal no other cause for her AF apart from her known risk factors.

Deciding on treatment

The NICE care pathway for AF recommends the use of the stroke risk stratification tool as a means of determining the best therapeutic choice. Using this scale, Agnes lies in the high risk zone. This is means that she is at high risk of a stroke and therefore the guideline advises that she should be treated with warfarin, with a target INR of 2.5 (range 2.0 to 3.0).

Treating Agnes's AF will reduce the risk of complications, which include:

- Thromboembolic episodes leading to stroke
- New or worsening heart failure
- Sudden death

(Lip et al, 1995).

Other considerations which may need discussion with Agnes and her daughter, Carrie, include the fact that:

- Women with AF have a higher risk of subsequent stroke than men
- In a follow-up of the Framingham study, atrial fibrillation was independently associated with a 50-90% increase in the risk of death

Furthermore, people who have underlying heart disease as well as AF, have an increased risk of stroke and up to 20% of patients with atrial fibrillation and a history of stroke will have a second stroke within one year (Benjamin, 1998).

Warfarin treatment

Antithrombotic therapy with warfarin should therefore be started as soon as is safely possible. Agnes will need to have the risks and benefits of treatment carefully explained to her prior to the initiation of therapy. According to the BAFTA trial (Mant et al, 2007), which looked at warfarin versus aspirin in stroke prevention for the over-75 age group, anticoagulation with warfarin will significantly reduce the risk of thromboembolic events for Agnes without increasing the risk of major bleeding. According to BAFTA, 50 patients need to be treated for one year to prevent one significant stroke. Therefore, it should be possible to explain that warfarin confers clear benefits with no real increase in the risk of major bleeding.

People with AF who are under the age of 75 can be managed with aspirin alone (75-300mg) as this has been shown to reduce the risk of stroke by 20%. Bandolier **(www.jr2.ox.ac.uk/bandolier)** suggests that in terms of numbers needed to treat (NNT), 48 patients would need to take aspirin for 18 months in order to prevent one stroke. It is important to remember, though, that all patients with AF who have any other risk factor (hypertension, ventricular dysfunction, valvular heart disease, previous history of thromboembolism) should be considered for anticoagulation with warfarin regardless of age. The BAFTA trial delivers further evidence to support this.

Anticoagulation clinics in primary care

Many practices are now running anticoagulation clinics, which minimises the inconvenience for patients like Agnes as the service is convenient and close to home. Tests may be undertaken fairly frequently at first but can to be performed less often as time goes on. The International Normalised Ratio (INR) blood test is used to monitor the effect of warfarin on coagulation. A target INR of 2.5 should be aimed for in Agnes's case but a range of between 2 and 3 is acceptable. The risk of bleeds increases steeply once the INR exceeds 3. Women have a higher risk of bleeding on warfarin than men but regular monitoring should help to ensure that all patients stay within safe limits.

If the INR changes unexpectedly, consider the following:

Raised INR:

◆ New carcinoma

◆ Increased alcohol intake

- Drug interactions with warfarin (see below)

- Taking too much warfarin (intentionally or accidentally)

- Reduced intake of vitamin K containing foods

- Acute diarrhoeal illness

- Taking more than 5 x 500mg paracetamol tablets per day (Bell, 1998)

Reduced INR:

- Increased intake of vitamin K in foods or supplements

Further management

The treatment strategy decision tree from NICE highlights the need for rate or rhythm control strategies based on the type of AF that Agnes has. We can divide AF into three main categories: Paroxysmal, Persistent, and Permanent AF.

- Paroxysmal AF resolves spontaneously within seven days, although most cases will resolve within 48 hours. It is recurrent. A third of patients with paroxysmal atrial fibrillation develop persistent or permanent AF over a period of two to three years. It is important, then, to identify and treat AF effectively at an early stage, especially as many sufferers will be asymptomatic

- Persistent AF is defined as AF which lasts longer than seven days and does not resolve spontaneously

- Permanent AF is that which continues or recurs after treatment.

Agnes can only say that she has been feeling below par for 'a few days'. Her notes reveal several recordings of a pulse rate over 90 bpm when her blood pressure has been measured, but none of them make reference to the rhythm. It is therefore not possible to be certain as to how long her atrial fibrillation has lasted. Nonetheless, the decision tree suggests that people over 65 may benefit primarily from rate control aimed at reducing the resting heart rate to less than 90. Overall, however, the choice of further treatment should then be made on an individual basis and in consultation with the patient.

Rate and rhythm controlling therapies

Beta blockers can be used to control both rate and rhythm and are often used in the management of AF. Other drugs used to control heart rate include rate limiting calcium channel blockers and digoxin, although this is generally used as add-in therapy if needed. Specialist drugs such as amiodarone may also be required. Treatments aimed at controlling rhythm include specialist drugs such as amiodarone, sotalol or flecainide.

Cardioversion

Cardioversion can be used to 'shock' the heart back into sinus rhythm. The INR must be stable for at least three weeks prior to this intervention. Anticoagulants are usually continued for at least four weeks following cardioversion and will be continued long term for patients at high risk of recurrence and stroke. Patients who are unsuitable for cardioversion include those not on anticoagulation therapy, those with some forms of structural heart disease, those whose AF is of over 12 month's duration and those with a history of previous unsuccessful attempts at cardioversion.

Referral criteria from primary care

Agnes should be referred to a cardiologist if drug treatment fails or if she requires cardioversion.

References

Bell WR (1998) Acetaminophen and warfarin. Undesirable synergy. *JAMA* 279:202-3

Benjamin ET et al (1998). Impact of atrial fibrillation on the risk of death. The Framingham Heart Study. *Circulation* 98:946-52

Cox, Beverley. Atrial fibrillation: giving your patients the best care. *British Journal of Primary Care Nursing – Cardiovascular Disease and Diabetes*, Volume 5, Issue 1 January-February 2008 Pages 42-46. *www.bjpcn-cardiovascular.com*

Hobbs FDR, Fitzmaurice DA, Mant J et al (2005) The SAFE study Health Technology Assesment 9:40

Kannel WB, Wolf PA, Benjamin EJ et al (1998) Prevalence, incidence, prognosis and predisposing conditions for atrial fibrillation: population based estimates. *American Journal of Cardiology* 82(8A):2N-9N

Lip GYH et al. (1995). The investigation and non-drug management of atrial fibrillation. *BMJ*, 311, 1562-5

Mant J et al (2007) Birmingham Atrial Fibrillation Treatment of the Aged. *Lancet* 370:493-503, 460-461

Ruigómez A et al. (2002) Incidence of chronic atrial fibrillation in general practice and its treatment pattern. *Journal of Clinical Epidemiology* 55: 358-363

Further information

www.arrhythmiaalliance.org.uk – the website of the organisation for patients and healthcare professionals with information on all types of heart arrhythmia

www.jr2.ox.ac.uk/bandolier - Bandolier: Evidence based healthcare in plain English *www.educationforhealth.org.uk* for information on diploma level courses in atrial fibrillation and stroke

www.gpnotebook.co.uk – free, evidence based website for general practice

www.mkupdate.co.uk for courses on understanding ECGs

www.nice.org.uk - for evidence based guidelines on AF

Chapter 8

Case study 12: Davina

Davina is a 49-year old woman who lives alone. She runs her own business as a complementary therapist and works part time. She came to the surgery complaining of feeling tired and run down, which she puts down to having candida. When asked to explain what she means by this she reports that she suffers from recurrent vaginal thrush which she treats with yoghurt and probiotics. Although this treatment appears to clear the thrush up she finds that it quickly recurs.

She did not attend the surgery very often as she preferred to treat herself but she was getting fed up of the thrush and had resorted to using diflucan and clotrimazole without success. A read through her records revealed that a blood test done three years ago when she also complained of tiredness had revealed a fasting blood glucose of 6.8mmol/L. A note had been put on the records asking her to come in to discuss this but she had not done so.

Davina's blood glucose level three years ago was sufficiently high to warrant investigations for possible impaired glucose tolerance. This would have meant that she had a glucose tolerance test to see how her body coped with a glucose load, delivered in a sugary drink. Bloods taken before and after the drink would indicate whether she was at risk of diabetes. Unfortunately, she had not attended for this test. The result and the implications of the previous test were explained to Davina, along with the need to repeat the blood glucose now.

Davina did not smoke and followed a vegetarian diet. She was also quite active. However, she was overweight with a BMI of 34 with a waist of 106cm. She reported that her father had been diagnosed with diabetes in his late 50s and had suffered from renal failure as a result. This had meant that she had been too anxious to come in for follow-up of her previous tests and had hoped to improve her general health through meditation.

The GP explained that meditation was an excellent way of ensuring an holistic approach to good health and that further interventions would ensure that her physical well being was as adequately cared for as her emotional well being. Subsequent blood tests revealed that Davina had unfortunately developed type 2 diabetes. The GP suggested a three-month period of careful attention to diet and activity levels and a review was arranged to measure the long term blood glucose control with a glycated haemoglobin level in three months time. In the meantime, Davina was encouraged to access the website of Diabetes UK so that she could read up on the evidence behind some of the therapies for diabetes and in particular, the need to view diabetes as a threat to her cardiovascular health. The HbA1c three months later was found to be 8.4% and after careful consideration of the options, Davina agreed to start on metformin for both its hypoglycaemic action and its cardioprotective action. Davina was then referred to the nurse practitioner for further advice and management.

Davina's bloods had also revealed a typical diabetic dyslipidaemia with a total cholesterol of 7.4mmol, an HDL-C of 0.9mmol and a triglyceride level of 2.9mmol. This is a potentially atherogenic profile: the high total cholesterol to HDL-C ratio of 8.2 means that the reverse transport mechanism whereby HDL-C removes cholesterol from the body is inefficient.

Davina was initially reluctant to consider a statin but eventually agreed, as she was anxious that she may end up like her father, exhibiting the cardiovascular 'fall-out' of diabetes.

Case study 13: Naz

Naz, aged 52, came in for a cholesterol test. He was keen to lose some weight as he has recently joined a gym and is embarrassed about his beer belly. He also thought that being overweight may have meant that he had a high cholesterol level and this worried him, as his brother-in-law had recently had a heart attack and the hospital had mentioned something about Asian men being at particularly high risk. He was currently being treated for hypertension with ramipril 5mg (in line with the British Hypertension Society/NICE guidelines) and he just started buying aspirin over the counter as he heard this was good for you. His blood test showed a cholesterol of 5.2mmol, an HDL-C of 0.7mmol and triglycerides of 1.9mmol. His BP is 132/84.

Naz's hypertension seems to be well controlled on ramipril 5mg and it would be easy to give some dietary advice and recommendations regarding exercise and send him on his way. However, from his history it would appear that he has a collection of risk factors for impaired glucose tolerance, metabolic syndrome, diabetes and cardiovascular disease. These include central obesity, previously diagnosed hypertension and his dyslipidaemia. Measuring his waist you discovered that it was 106cm – confirming his increased risk of all of these conditions.

In order to assess his glycaemic state the doctor ordered a fasting blood glucose and this is reported as being 6.2mmol. Diabetes is diagnosed when the fasting blood glucose is >7mmol, so this result would not fall into that category. However, neither was the result normal, as it is above 6.1mmol. Therefore, Naz may have abnormal glucose metabolism, with all of the inherent risks that come with that condition. So how should he be managed?

The nurse practitioner decided to get a glucose tolerance test done. Doing a GTT meant that instead of just getting a snapshot of Naz's glucose level at any given time it was possible to see how his body coped when going from a fasting state to dealing with a glucose load. The GTT confirmed a diagnosis of impaired glucose tolerance (IGT), another marker for metabolic syndrome.

There is good evidence to suggest that IGT will respond to lifestyle changes. Losing weight, becoming more active and increasing muscle mass will impact on the way in which the body metabolises glucose. It was important for Naz to understand that these recommendations do not just amount to the usual 'lose weight, take more exercise' mantra that healthcare professionals are prone to trot out at every opportunity; for Naz this advice is based on improving the way in which his body carries out glucose metabolism in the future. For instance, Naz needs to understand that building up muscle will help to increase the amount of sugar that is removed from the blood stream by those muscles, thus reducing the tendency to hyperglycaemia. Some clinicians may also decide to initiate medication to reduce the risk of developing diabetes. Drugs which have been shown to be useful include metformin, acarbose and possibly the glitazones. Ramipril may also reduce the risk of diabetes.

Diabetes is a cardiotoxic time bomb and it is important that clinicians understand their duty to reduce cardiovascular risk in all of their patients with diabetes. In 2008, Diabetes UK reviewed the progress being made in diabetes care since the National Service Framework began. Their report stated that:

"For the majority of people, then, this will include giving some or all of the following drugs:

◆ Metformin – to reduce blood glucose levels and provide cardiovascular protection

◆ ACE inhibitors – for the 75%+ of people with diabetes who also have hypertension

◆ Aspirin – to people with diabetes over the age of 50, unless their overall risk is thought to be low

◆ Statin – to reduce CVD risk"

Some people think that all of these drugs could be packed together into one easy to take tablet, known as the 'polypill'!

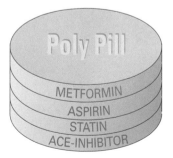

JAMA.2006; 296: 377-380

Managing lipid levels in high risk patients

In 1961 the Framingham Heart Study (**www.framinghamheartstudy.org**) showed that raised cholesterol levels contribute to the risk of developing heart disease and 17 years later in 1988 the link between low HDL-C levels and heart disease was established via the same study. Statin therapy is the first line treatment for dyslipidaemia with simvastatin 40mg being the recommended drug in terms of cost efficacy (NICE 2008a), whether treatment is being given for primary or secondary prevention.

In primary prevention, ie where there is no evidence of established cardiovascular disease but where the 10-year risk has been assessed as being over 20%, NICE recommends a 'fire and forget' strategy. This means that there is no lipid target to be reached – the only target is to get patients onto statin therapy in order to reduce their risk.

However, in high risk patients, where there is already evidence of CVD, or in patients with diabetes where the CVD risk is thought to be equivalent to someone who has already had an event, a more intensive approach to managing lipids is needed.

Case study 14: Rita

Rita is a 53 year old lady with type 1 diabetes. She was diagnosed aged three and has already shown evidence of retinopathy and nephropathy. In her 30s she was also diagnosed with rheumatoid arthritis. Her lipid profile is atherogenic with an LDL-C of 4.2mmol. She has tried simvastatin 40mg previously but found that she suffered side effects, including myalgia and indigestion at night after taking it. Her bloods did not indicate any underlying reason for this but she was reluctant to continue with her statin and the subject had not been raised again for the past year.

At her annual review, however, the practice nurse once again initiated discussion around the benefits of statin therapy, highlighting the high level of risk that both her diabetes and her RA posed in terms of CVD. After careful discussion about the possible options, Rita decided to try rosuvastatin 10mg as it has been shown to be effective in reducing lipid levels and is often acceptable to people who have not previously been able to tolerate other statins. This is because rosuvastatin, along with the weaker pravastatin, is metabolised differently from the other statins. Rosuvastatin can also be taken at any time of day, thus reducing the risk of night-time indigestion.

Case study 15: Jake

Jake is a 72 year old man who has had a myocardial infarction in the past. In patients who have been diagnosed with acute coronary syndrome, like Jake, there is evidence to suggest that the use of high intensity statins should be standard practice (NICE 2008a). Target lipid levels should be a total cholesterol of <4mmol and an LDL-C of <2mmol. Following his MI, Jake was started on atorvastatin 80mg. At his annual review in the GP surgery, Jake's lipids were noted to be as follows:

- ◆ TC 4.6mmol

- ◆ HDL 1.0mmol

- ◆ LDL 2.2mmol

Once concordance had been established, the decision had to be made regarding 2nd line treatment of this lipid profile. Options include switching to another high intensity statin (rosuvastatin) and/or adding further drugs which might complement the action of the statin, using ezetimibe, adding a fibrate, using a nicotinic acid preparation to increase the HDL-C or introducing bile acid sequestrants, e.g. cholestyramine. After discussion with Jake it was decided to add ezetimibe 10mg once daily to complement the action of the atorvastatin.

Case study 16: Mick

Mick is 31 and attended the surgery after suffering an episode of chest pain on two occasions after running on the treadmill at the gym. He was a bit worried as his father had died of a heart attack in his late 40s. He had never attended a GP surgery in his adult life but admitted that this episode had frightened him. Initial measurements showed a BP of 134/88 and a BMI of 35, although Mick was a regular gym goer and did weight training five times a week – his physique was quite muscular but his waist measurement was 98cm, indicating central obesity. He was referred to the Rapid Access Chest Pain Clinic and was prescribed aspirin 75mg daily and a GTN spray to take should the pain recur. In the meantime he was asked to have blood tests done. When the results came through they showed that Mick's total cholesterol was 13.9mmol, his HDL-C was 1.1mmol, with triglycerides of 3.8mmol. His ratio was 12.6 and his LDL-C was 11.1mmol. His thyroid function tests were normal as was his blood glucose, liver function and renal function. This lipid profile fits the criteria for a diagnosis of familial hypercholesterolaemia (FH) (NICE 2008b).

FH is a genetic condition which results in raised levels of LDL-C from birth, leading to premature development of CVD. Siblings and children of a person with FH have a 50% risk of inheriting FH themselves. The clinical diagnosis of FH is made using the Simon Broome criteria, as defined in the NICE guidance (see Table 8.2). The diagnosis can be confirmed using DNA testing which will be carried out following referral to a specialist in lipid disorders. People with FH should have cascade tracing of relatives who may be affected.

Table 8.1: Cholesterol levels to be used as diagnostic criteria for the index individual *Marks D, Thorogood M, Neil HA, Humphries SE (2003) A review on the diagnosis, natural history, and treatment of familial hypercholesterolaemia. Atherosclerosis 168 (1): 1-14.*

	Total Cholesterol	LDL-C:
Adult	>7.5 mmol/l	>4.9 mmol/l
Child	>6.7 mmol/l	>4.0 mmol/l

Levels either pre-treatment or highest on treatment

Table 8.2: The Simon Broome criteria for diagnosing familial hypercholesterolaemia

Diagnose a person with DEFINITE FH if they have:

◆ Cholesterol concentrations as above and tendon xanthomas, or evidence of these signs in first or second-degree relative

or

◆ DNA-based evidence of an LDL-receptor mutation, familial defective apo B-100, or a PCSK9 mutation.

Diagnose a person with POSSIBLE FH if they have cholesterol concentrations as defined above and at least one of the following:

◆ Family history of myocardial infarction: aged younger than 50 years in second-degree relative or aged younger than 60 years in first-degree relative.

◆ Family history of raised total cholesterol: greater than 7.5 mmol/l in adult first or second-degree relative, or greater than 6.7 mmol/l in child, brother or sister aged younger than 16 years.

In line with NICE guidance, and under specialist supervision, Mick was offered treatment with the maximum dose of a high intensity statin, which for him was rosuvastatin 40mg, and ezetimibe 10mg. Further treatment was also needed and he was given cholestyramine 12g daily. He remains under the care of the lipidologist for his lipid problems and his two daughters, age 10 and 12 are also being followed up, along with other members of his family. He is also undergoing follow-up with the cardiology team as he has been confirmed as having triple vessel disease, which was causing angina. Primary care had a vital role in picking up this man and identifying the risk both to him and to his family. He will need ongoing care from both primary and secondary care for the foreseeable future.

References

Cox, Beverley. Impaired Fasting Glycaemia and Impaired Glucose Tolerance: Reducing Progression. *British Journal of Primary Care Nursing – Cardiovascular Disease and Diabetes*, Volume 5, Number 2, March-April 2008 *www.bjpcn-cardiovascular.com*

NICE Lipid Modification guideline CG67 (2008a) available from www.nice.org.uk/CG067

NICE (2008b) Familial hypercholesterolaemia: NICE guideline CG71 available from *www.nice.org.uk/guidance/index.jsp?action=download&o=41698*

Case study 17: Enid

Enid was on the caseload of the district nursing team as she had Lupus disease, complicated by occasional falls and intermittent problems with leg ulcers. She tried very hard to be as independent as possible, however, and so it was surprising when the team received a phone call from her requesting an extra visit as she was so breathless that she could not get out of her chair – it was that much effort. When the nurse arrived at Enid's home she found her to be much more breathless than normal and she was also looking oddly flushed across her jaw, although her temperature was normal. Other observations revealed a BP of 167/101, an irregular pulse of 116 and a respiratory rate of 36. There was evidence of ankle oedema, a palpable thrill and a possible murmur heard, which was more noticeable when Enid lay on her left side. However, lying down made her much more breathless.

In view of the fact that Enid was haemodynamically impaired, possibly because of atrial fibrillation, the district nurse arranged for Enid to be admitted to hospital. Further examination there revealed the presence of a raised JVP and a chest X-ray showed possible enlargement of the atria. An echo was ordered which confirmed the diagnosis of severe mitral stenosis. Enid was stabilised prior to surgical repair of her mitral valve.

Enid presented with a range of acute cardio-respiratory symptoms which could have been caused by a range of diseases. When working in primary care, however, it is important in an acute situation such as Enid's to seek further advice regarding assessment, diagnosis and management as soon as possible once the initial assessment has alerted the clinician to the possibility of life-threatening illness.

Peripheral Arterial Disease (PAD), also known as Peripheral Vascular Disease (PVD), is a vascular condition which affects the legs. It is caused by atherosclerosis – narrowing and hardening of the arteries – and has previously been described as being similar to angina in the legs. Sufferers get cramping pains in their legs when they walk, which is relieved by rest; this is similar to the chest pain that coronary heart disease (CHD) patients get. The similarities between CHD and PAD do not end there: not only are the symptoms similar but the causes and the treatments overlap, too. This chapter will explain how three patients presenting in surgery with symptoms suggestive of PAD were treated.

Case study 18: Geoff

Geoff is a 54 year old lorry driver who lives locally. He presents with a history of cramp in his legs after he has been driving for long distances. He comes to see you to see if you can prescribe him 'some cramp tablets', as he thinks that these will help.

What would you do?

Geoff's 'cramp' may well be intermittent claudication caused by PAD. The pain he describes could be caused by a the sudden increase in the amount of oxygen needed by the tissues in his legs when he gets out of his cab and starts moving around. Although it is important not to 'pigeon-hole' patients, it is worth checking Terry's lifestyle and health behaviours if he works as a lorry driver. This occupation may well involve long periods of inactivity while driving followed by bursts of activity when Geoff arrives at his destination and has to unload his lorry.

Driving is also a stressful activity. Lorry drivers may also tend to eat less healthily and smoke more owing to the amount of time they spend on the road. In line with the current recommendations from the government, then, Geoff needs a full cardiovascular risk assessment. It turns out that Geoff's blood pressure is raised at 161/96 on this occasion, even after you have checked it three times. He needs a full review and some bloods doing in order to assess his cardiovascular risk. The good news is that he stopped smoking six years ago and you make a point of congratulating Geoff regarding this.

Testing for Peripheral Arterial Disease[1]

Manual palpation of the femoral, popliteal and pedal pulses can serve as an indication of the state of the peripheral vessels. It is important to remember, however, that it is possible to have PAD, even if the pulses are palpable.

In the case of someone like Geoff, who has possible symptoms of PAD, objective tests will be needed. This usually involves measuring the Ankle Brachial Pressure Index (ABPI) in both legs. This test should not be used in people with diabetes or chronic renal failure as it is unreliable due to possible calcification of the vessels. ABPI measurement involves the use of a sphygmomanometer and a hand held Doppler device. This requires training but there are many practitioners in primary care, and in particular in district nursing teams, who are competent and well practised in this area if you are unable to do it yourself.

Table 10.1: Understanding ABPI results

If ABPI is >0.9 this is considered to be normal

Resting ABPI is <0.9 in 95% cases of PAD, including asymptomatic disease

ABPI is 0.5-0.9 in most patients with intermittent claudication

ABPI <0.5 indicates more severe disease, including critical ischaemia

If ABPI is normal but the patient has symptoms – refer

If ABPI is 1.5+ the reading is unlikely to be reliable – refer to secondary care for further assessment

NB: The lower the ABPI the greater the risk of future cardiovascular events

A useful guide to measuring ABPI is available as part of the PAD guideline on the SIGN website[2].

Visit two

Geoff misses his review in two weeks but turns up two weeks after that apologising for the delay, which was due to work commitments. You take time to explain to him that these appointments are really important if he is to take care of his heart and that it's great that he has made sure to come back. His BP this time is 156/94. His bloods show that his lipids are abnormal with a total cholesterol of 7.2mmol, HDL of 0.9mmol and triglycerides of 2.2mmol. He also has a fasting glucose of 6.1mmol, which is not in the range suggesting diabetes but is certainly in the possible range for impaired fasting glycaemia. Other bloods, including renal and hepatic function, a full blood count and thyroid function tests are all normal. You decide to arrange a glucose tolerance test to assess the standard of Geoff's glucose metabolism.

Visit three

On this occasion Geoff's BP is 159/93 and you decide that a diagnosis of hypertension is now justified. Geoff is quite worried about all of these tests as his father died of a coronary at 64. He had suffered three previous heart attacks before the one that killed him, too. You are beginning to share Geoff's concern! Geoff's family history needs to be taken into account when assessing his risk. The fact that he has hypertension, impaired fasting glycaemia – as confirmed on his GTT – and dyslipidaemia, means that his risk is elevated.

Visit four

Geoff is very anxious about the results of his risk assessment. His ABPI is 0.9 which just puts him into the abnormal range, suggesting PAD. He is therefore now known to be at increased CVD risk as he already has evidence of vascular disease in his legs. Geoff will therefore need to make changes to his lifestyle and health behaviours, as well as having pharmacological treatment for his risk factors. The drugs recommended for Geoff will be the same as those used in managing CHD: statins, anti-hypertensive therapies and aspirin 75mg. If aspirin cannot be tolerated, clopidogrel can be substituted. There is some evidence that the use of ACE inhibitors can be particularly beneficial in PAD[3]. Although exercise has been shown to be beneficial in people with PAD, care is needed in view of the symptoms. Nonetheless, exercise should be encouraged within reason.

Treating intermittent claudication

There are few effective treatments for the symptoms of PAD and some that are effective have a high side effect profile, which makes them difficult for patients to tolerate. The most commonly used drug is the vasodilator naftidrofuryl, which is usually taken three times a day, thus leading to possible concordance issues. Another drug, cilostazol, has also been licensed for intermittent claudication due to PAD, and can be used if other therapies have been unsuccessful.

Annual review

People like Geoff, who have PAD, are at increased risk of suffering a cardiovascular event, such as a stroke or heart attack, and have higher cardio-vascular mortality rates than those with CHD or other forms of CVD[4]. Geoff will need to be reviewed at least annually and will need a full assessment of his symptoms, lifestyle and drug therapies. In cases of severe or worsening symptoms it is important to refer for a surgical opinion. Although there is limited evidence of benefit of surgery in patients with intermittent claudication, it is vital that people with more severe symptoms are seen by a vascular surgeon for a surgical opinion.

Case study 19: Jas

Jas, age 59, presents with tiredness, which has been present for the past three months. She is an overweight Asian lady, with a BMI of 28. She has little enthusiasm for watching her diet and taking more exercise, which is what you advised when you saw her in your weight management clinic six months ago, and she has not made any significant changes in her health behaviours since then apart from drinking more water. What might be the problem with Jas?

You decide to check Jas's bloods as you are suspicious that she may have type 2 diabetes. Her bloods confirm that this is so. However, on further questioning you discover that her reluctance to exercise is compounded by the fact that she has symptoms of PAD – specifically intermittent claudication. Jas will need a full review and assessment of her lifestyle, drug therapy and ABPI measurements, just as you did with Terry. You are aware that ABPI measurements are not as reliable in people with diabetes so decide to refer to the joint diabetes and vascular team for a thorough peripheral vascular assessment.

PAD is an important vascular condition, causing significant morbidity and mortality but which may currently be overlooked by clinicians. People with PAD can benefit from the range of interventions routinely offered to patients with CHD and stroke, but this is not always recognised. It is vital, then, that primary care nurses are aware of the possibility of PAD, including the symptoms of intermittent claudication, when assessing people for both cardiovascular risk and evidence of overt disease. Once identified, PAD should be treated with the same degree of importance as CHD already is.

References

1. Cox, Beverley. Hands on peripheral arterial disease. *British Journal of Primary Care Nursing – Cardiovascular Disease and Diabetes*, Volume 5, Issue 4 July-August 2008 Pages 181- 183. www.bjpcn-cardiovascular.com

2. Scottish Intercollegiate Guidelines Network (SIGN) (2006) Guideline 89: Peripheral Arterial Disease (PAD). Access at www.sign.ac.uk

3. Ostergren J, Sleight P, Dagenais G et al (2004) Impact of ramipril in patients with evidence of clinical or sub clinical peripheral arterial disease. *European Heart Journal* 25: 17-24

4. Steg GL et al. (2007) One-year cardiovascular event rates in outpatients with atherothrombosis. *JAMA* 297:1197-206

Further information

www.targetpad.co.uk/index.aspx Target PAD – a website run by healthcare professionals dedicated to improving PAD care

www.gpnotebook.co.uk General advice on a range of subjects

www.patient.co.uk Advice for patients

www.bhf.org.uk British Heart Foundation website

www.tasc-pad.org/html/index.html The TransAtlantic Inter-Society (TASC) guidelines on PAD

www.educationforhealth.org.uk Information on courses on CVD Risk Assessment, CHD, Stroke, Hypertension and Diabetes as a Cardiovascular Disease

We have already touched on the importance of risk assessment for CVD in various groups of the population. However, the government's document 'Putting Prevention First' (DH 2008) suggests that all people between the ages of 40 and 75 should be screened for cardiovascular risk and that those people found to have a risk score of 20% or more should be treated. This can be challenging for the clinician, who may have to persuade a patient to take a statin, for instance, every day for the rest of their life to prevent an event which might never happen!

Case study 20: Mary

Mary is 54 years old and has a family history of CVD, with her father suffering his first heart attack in his 50s. Bloods revealed an interesting lipid profile: TC 7.1, HDL 0.7 and triglycerides of 6.2. Her risk assessment score was 24% and she clearly needed treatment. She was started on 40mg of simvastatin and was given the following patient information leaflet:

Starting on your statin for primary prevention[1]

What is this pill for?

Statins are a treatment to lower your cholesterol level.

Why am I being advised to take it?

Lower cholesterol levels have been shown to reduce your chance of having a heart attack or stroke in the future. Based on your current level of risk, you are likely to benefit from lowering your cholesterol.

What is a healthy cholesterol level?

A cholesterol level of 5 or less is good with levels of 4 or less being ideal. However, there are different types of cholesterol (lipids) and the ratio of good cholesterol to bad cholesterol is also important.

What dose should I take?

Guidelines from the National Institute of Health and Clinical Excellence (NICE) recommend the use of simvastatin 40mg as this has been shown to be highly effective in the majority of people. If this is not suitable for any reason, then an alternative may be prescribed.

When should I take it?

Some cholesterol comes from your food but it is important to realise that your body also makes its own cholesterol in your liver. Most of this cholesterol is made at night-time so you may get more benefit if you take your tablet at night-time too. Talk to your doctor, nurse or pharmacist if you think this may be difficult for any reason.

How will I know it is working?

Studies have shown that simvastatin 40mg reduces the risk of heart attacks and strokes in most of the people who take it. For this reason there is no need to have routine blood tests to look at your lipid levels once you have started on your tablet. However, your liver function will be tested at three and 12 months to ensure that the drug is suiting you.

How long should I take it for?

Your cholesterol level will be lowered by taking the tablets. If you stop taking them, your cholesterol will rise again. For this reason we advise that you should keep taking the tablets for as long as possible and ideally for life.

What side effects might I expect and how common are they?

Side effects from statins are surprisingly rare. However, all drugs have side effects – even 'dummy' pills used in medical trials have been shown to cause side effects in some people, so it is not always the tablet that is to blame. With statins, rare side effects include muscle pains and indigestion and you should let your doctor, nurse or pharmacist know if these occur. It is important to remember, however, that the likely benefits from statins are greater than the risks for the vast majority of people.

What if I decide that I do not want to take these pills?

Your doctor or nurse will have advised you to take these tablets because you are likely to benefit from reducing your risk of a heart attack or stroke. High cholesterol does not make you feel unwell so it can sometimes be hard to understand why you should take a tablet for the rest of your life. Nonetheless, it is worth remembering that huge medical trials have proven the benefit of these pills in reducing the risk of heart attack or stroke.

Is there an alternative?

You can and should try to eat healthily. Taking regular exercise such as walking can raise your 'good' cholesterol. You should also try to lose weight if you need to. Taking statins will ADD to these changes. Mildly raised cholesterol can be improved by diet and exercise but studies show that statins will lower the levels further.

Is there any harm in lowering my cholesterol? Can my cholesterol go too low?

Statins have been used for over 30 years and no significant long term problems have been shown in any of the trials. Recent trials have looked at lowering cholesterol levels to 3 or less, and overall it seems the lower the level the less the risk of heart attacks and strokes.

Any other questions?

Talk to your doctor, nurse or pharmacist, or go to **www.heartuk.org.uk**

Mary has had no side effects from her statin and has exhorted her siblings to have their lipid profiles checked. It may well be that Mary has a mixed familial hyperlipidaemia and she was referred to the GPwSI in lipid management for further follow-up. A simple algorithm for statin initiation follows:

Table 11.1: Initiating statins

Check liver function tests to ensure that they are normal prior to commencing the statin. Use this opportunity to check for any possible cause for dyslipidaemia such as hypothyroidism or undiagnosed diabetes – check thyroid function tests and blood glucose measurement

In line with NICE guidelines, start patient on simvastatin 40mg and give repeat blood form

After six weeks, repeat lipid profile and liver function tests. Only measure creatine kinase (CK) if the patient is suffering from muscle pain (myalgia).

If LFTs (or creatinine kinase) have risen, repeat bloods in another six weeks

Uptitrate the statin if necessary, in accordance with NICE guidelines. In primary prevention, there is no target level. In secondary prevention, or in patients with diabetes, aim for target lipid levels of 4mmol total cholesterol or less or 2mmol low density lipoprotein or less, as per NICE guidance, although interim targets (also referred to as audit targets) can be aimed for initially – these are total cholesterol of 5mmol and LDL of 3mmol.

If target levels are not achieved, increase the dose of simvastatin to 80mg or consider using alternative statins, such as atorvastatin or rosuvastatin, especially if side effects are an issue. Alternatively, consider adding in a drug to complement the statin, such as ezetimibe, a fibrate or nicotinic acid.

References

1. Cox, Beverley. Starting on a statin for primary prevention. *British Journal of Primary Care Nursing – Cardiovascular Disease and Diabetes,* Volume 5, Issue 6 November-December 2008 Page 299. *www.bjpcn-cardiovascular.com*

Chapter 12

Hands-on INR – understanding INR and warfarin

With the advent of guidelines from NICE regarding the management of conditions such as Atrial Fibrillation (NICE, 2006) and the publication of research evidence from trials such as the Birmingham Atrial Fibrillation Treatment of the Aged Study (Mant et al, 2007) the use of warfarin is becoming more widespread and the drug is perhaps being seen as the lifesaver that it is, rather than something to be avoided unless absolutely necessary.

More and more nurses in primary care will be involved in monitoring INR levels and advising patients on warfarin doses as anticoagulation clinics move out of secondary care and into primary care. It is vital that practice nurses are also aware of possible interactions between warfarin and other drugs which might be prescribed by the nurse, such as statins or antibiotics. They also need to be able to advise on lifestyle interventions which go hand in hand with taking warfarin.

Warfarin was developed back in the 1950s from the sweet clover plant after it was observed that cows that ate lots of sweet clover developed bleeding problems. Approximately one million people in the UK now take warfarin.

Case study 21: Katherine

Katherine comes to see you in surgery. She is a 78 year old retired school teacher who has a history of hypertension. She has been treated with ramipril 10mg, bendroflumethiazide 2.5mg and amlodipine 5mg for several years. Her last blood pressure reading four months ago was 142/78. Three weeks ago she had an episode of acute breathlessness and chest pain at the weekend and was admitted to hospital as an emergency, where she was diagnosed as having atrial fibrillation (AF). Katherine has always had her own ideas about how to manage her hypertension. She has now been started on warfarin but as she knows you well, wants to discuss the pros and cons of the treatment and the monitoring. She hates blood tests!

How would you explain the role of warfarin in AF to Katherine?

In order to understand what warfarin is doing and the significance of blood testing, we need to clarify how the normal clotting process works and how warfarin interacts with this process.

Many substances are involved in clotting, one of which is prothrombin. As its name suggests, prothrombin is used to enable clots to develop. This is vital in times of injury but can be counterproductive in cases where the blood needs to be kept 'thinner' so that it flows more easily and is less likely to clot and block up a vessel. The prothrombin time (PT) is a measure of how long it takes for the blood to clot and is assessed by mixing a sample of blood with a reagent and the number of seconds taken for the blood to clot is counted. Different reagents are used by different laboratories for this test, so the result is then translated into a standardised range known as the International Normalised Ratio (INR).

All INR measurements are measured against the normal value for someone whose blood clotting status is healthy and who is not taking any anticoagulant medication. This normal value is 1. If the blood takes longer to clot than normal, the INR will be higher, as the number of seconds before clotting occurs will increase. The lower the INR value, the more likely the blood is to clot quicker; the higher the INR value, the longer the blood will take to clot. It is obvious then, that INR values must not go too high or the risk of bleeding will outweigh the benefits of anticoagulation.

Some people need warfarin because they have an increased risk of clots developing, either because they have already suffered from an abnormal clotting event such as a thrombosis; others need warfarin because they suffer from a condition where clots are more likely to occur leading to further health problems. In Katherine's case her atrial fibrillation means that the heart beat is irregular, allowing tiny clots to develop within the heart which can then travel up to the brain causing a stroke. AF is a strong risk factor for stroke (Wolf et al, 1991). Keeping the blood thinner will reduce the risk of clots being allowed to develop within the heart and will therefore reduce Katherine's risk of a stroke in the future *(Lip et al, 2006)*.

As warfarin interferes with the clotting process, careful monitoring of the INR will be needed to ensure that she reaps the benefits of the drug without increasing her risk of bleeding unnecessarily. This monitoring is carried out by checking the INR measurement on a regular basis and keeping it within the recommended target range for her condition. All of this information will be recorded in her Yellow Book, which will also include advice on her target INR and her recommended dose regime. The Yellow Book is retained by the patient in between visits to the anticoagulation clinic, and is a useful resource for other clinicians.

Target ranges for INR will vary according to the condition being treated but for most conditions, the INR target range will be 2 to 3.5. An INR above 5 is potentially dangerous as the risk of bleeding increases significantly above this level.

Katherine was very interested to hear about the way in which lifestyle and other medication being taken over the counter could impact on her INR. Her friend had been taking warfarin and had been told that she must avoid alcohol as this was likely to lead to a rise in her INR. Katherine was not sure that she could contemplate a life without her daily glass of red! What would you advise her?

Factors that can influence the INR do indeed include alcohol. Others include diet, activity levels, prescribed and over the counter medication and herbal remedies. Alcohol should be avoided if possible when taking warfarin as it affects the way in which the drug is metabolised and may also increase the risk of gastric bleeds if drunk to excess. However, if Katherine wishes to have a glass of wine a day then this is acceptable as long as she keeps her intake low and steady and avoids overindulging. Cranberry and grapefruit juices are also thought to affect the metabolism of warfarin so should generally be avoided.

Vitamin K is important for the production of proteins involved in clotting. Warfarin works by preventing the body from using vitamin K effectively, thus reducing its clotting ability. Therefore, if Katherine's intake of vitamin K suddenly increases her warfarin dose may have to increase to counteract the extra vitamin K. Green leafy vegetables are a good source of vitamin K and Katherine has been trying to eat more healthily since her recent admission so this could possibly be something that needs to be borne in mind, especially if her good intentions fall by the wayside and she reverts to her previous dietary habits in a few weeks or months. The most important aspect of diet and lifestyle activities is that they are kept consistent, as it is the stability of the diet and lifestyle week by week that matters rather than small day to day alterations. Foods containing high levels of vitamin K should not be avoided, then, but Katherine should try to ensure that her intake of these foods remains stable from week to week.

Foods which have high levels of Vitamin K include:

◆ Spinach

◆ Broccoli

◆ Cabbage

◆ Lettuce

◆ Sprouts

◆ Watercress

Katherine should be reminded that any signs of bleeding should be monitored and reported. These would include any nose bleeds, bleeding from the gums and unprovoked or excessive bruising. More serious signs include haemoptysis, haematemesis or malaena.

Katherine phones you during afternoon surgery the following week to say that she has forgotten to take her warfarin that morning. What should you advise?

The action of warfarin lasts for several days so if a dose is accidentally omitted, or an extra dose is taken, the effect on the INR may be seen for several days, which is why care with taking the medication is so important. Concordance issues must always be considered with any drug, but maybe more so with warfarin. Used wisely it is a life-saver, but when misused it has the potential for grave side effects. Katherine needs to be aware of this and think about the best time of day for her to take it. Warfarin can be taken at any time of day, to suit the individual and their lifestyle. A missed dose may be taken up to 12 hours after the time it was due. An extra dose should be reported to the clinician, as further INR testing may be necessary. Any missed doses should be reported at the next INR test appointment. As it is less than 12 hours since Katherine missed her dose she can take it now and resume her usual routine from tomorrow.

Katherine had been on the internet and has read about home testing devices that can be used to provide a finger-prick sample which will measure the INR. She would like you to prescribe one for her. How would you respond to this request?

Home testing devices for INR are similar to home testing devices for blood glucose in that they are used in a similar way but are also not prescribable on the NHS. The device can be bought privately, however, at a cost usually in excess of £500. The testing strips can be prescribed, although some patients have had difficulty getting prescriptions from some Primary Care Trusts. Some anticoagulation clinics being run in the community use these devices to measure INR as they get an instant result. If the result is outside of the normal range the test can be repeated immediately to ensure that it is a true reading. All results can then be acted upon immediately and warfarin doses adjusted by the specialist clinician before the patient leaves the premises.

Case study 22: Suzanne

Suzanne is 28 years old and was very healthy until, out of the blue, she suffered from a deep vein thrombosis (DVT) after delivering her first child two years ago. She is now planning another pregnancy and requests your advice regarding restarting her warfarin. Her view is that she should take it to avoid another clot. What would you say?

Warfarin is normally continued for at least three months following a DVT, although this will vary from individual to individual, depending on their risk of further DVTs. Warfarin is contraindicated in pregnancy, however, as it is teratogenic. Suzanne needs referral for advice regarding the need for anticoagulation in her next pregnancy. If this is recommended then she will be treated with heparin, which is safe to use in pregnancy. The good news is that warfarin can be taken safely when breast feeding. The target INR for DVT is usually 2.5 with a range of 2 to 3.

Case study 23: Roger

Roger is 73 years old and has chronic left ventricular systolic dysfunction. He is on treatment with ramipril 10mg and furosemide 40mg. He initially tolerated the introduction of a beta blocker (bisoprolol) well, but then developed reversible airways disease and so it had to be stopped. After further assessment by his cardiologist he was referred for consideration of an implantable device. One month ago he was operated on and a biventricular pacemaker was implanted along with a defibrillator. He made a superb recovery and is now on warfarin. He comes into surgery because he has had a call from the laboratory to say that his INR is currently 6 and he must stop taking his warfarin immediately. He is extremely anxious.

What should you do?

You should check with Roger what his usual routine is for taking his warfarin in case he has inadvertently taken an extra dose, leading to his high INR. Also, is he taking another type of medication which may affect his INR? (See list below). Don't forget to include things he may have bought over the counter. Check his alcohol intake recently and remind him to keep his intake steady and avoid any binge drinking. Ask him about his general health – is he well or has he noticed any new symptoms or a possible exacerbation of an ongoing problem such as Chronic Obstructive Pulmonary Disease (COPD)? Finally, has he noticed any signs of bleeding (see above) which might indicate the need for further intervention? Any symptoms of significant bleeding, such as a gastro-intestinal bleed, are likely to require admission to hospital.

The usual advice in a case like this would be to stop the warfarin for 1-2 days and then recheck the INR.

The tables below show the drugs which interact with warfarin (from the CKS website – see resource list at end of chapter).

Table 12.1: Medications that *enhance* the effect of warfarin	
Prescribable medicines	OTC or non-conventional
Amiodarone	Alcohol
Aspirin (analgesic or antiplatelet use)	Aspirin or medicines containing aspirin
Corticosteroids, especially at high dose	Paracetamol / preparations containing paracetamol
Influenza vaccine	Cranberry juice
Macrolide antibiotics e.g. erythromycin	Grapefruit juice
Non-steroidal anti-inflammatory drugs	Glucosamine
Paracetamol	
Proton pump inhibitors	
Quinolone antibiotics e.g. ciprofloxacin	
Selective serotonin re-uptake inhibitors (SSRIs)	
Statins	
Thyroxine	

Table 12.2: Medications that *may reduce* the effect of warfarin

Prescribable medicines	Others
Carbamazepine	St John's Wort
Oral contraceptives	
Phenytoin	
Rifampicin	
Vitamin K	

Conclusion

More and more people need to take warfarin. In general, anticoagulation advice, including recommendations regarding doses of warfarin and frequency of INR testing should be given by clinicians with specific training in this area, whether anticoagulation clinics are held in primary or secondary care settings. However, nurses working in primary care must be aware of key issues such as target ranges for INR depending on the condition being treated, and drugs and lifestyle issues which might impact on the dose of warfarin needed or the frequency of blood tests. The patient's hand-held record, also known as the Yellow Book, will contain specific information about their target INR range, their current dosing regime and dates of their blood tests.

References

Cox, Beverley. Anticoagulation in Practice: Why it Matters that the Dose of Warfarin is Spot On. *British Journal of Primary Care Nursing – Cardiovascular Disease, Diabetes and Kidney Care*, Volume 6, Issue 2 April-June 2009 Pages 60-63. *www.bjpcn-cardiovascular.com*

Lip GY, Tello-Montoliu A (2006) Management of atrial fibrillation. *Heart* 92 (8):177–82

Mant J, Hobbs FD, Fletcher K, et al (2007) Warfarin versus aspirin for stroke prevention in an elderly community population with atrial fibrillation (the Birmingham Atrial Fibrillation Treatment of the Aged Study, BAFTA): a randomised controlled trial. *Lancet* 370(9586): 493-503

NICE clinical guideline 36 for Atrial Fibrillation (2006) Available from *www.nice.org.uk/Guidance/CG36*

Wolf PA, Abbott RD, Kannel WB (1991) Atrial fibrillation as an independent risk factor for stroke: the Framingham Study. *Stroke* 22 (8): 983–988.

Further resources

Anticoagulation Europe
PO Box 405, Bromley, Kent BR2 9WP
Tel: 020 8289 6875
Web: *www.anticoagulationeurope.org*

Arrhythmia Alliance
www.aral.org.uk/

Atrial fibrillation and warfarin available from
www.patient.co.uk/showdoc/23068883/

British Heart Foundation,
14 Fitzhardinge Street,
London W1H 6DH
Tel (Heart Help Line): 08450 70 80 70
Web: *www.bhf.org.uk*

Clinical Knowledge Summaries – evidence based guidelines from the NHS on a range of topics available from: *http://cks.library.nhs.uk/home*

CKS advice on drug interactions with warfarin. Advice available from: *http://cks.library.nhs.uk/atrial_fibrillation/management/quick_answers/ scenario_antithrombotic_treatment/which_therapy/ practical_prescribing_points/drug_interactions_with_warfarin*

In spite of the many cases covered so far, it is important to remember that not all cases of chest pain or breathlessness are caused by cardiovascular disorders. Key pointers away from cardiovascular disease are shown in Table 13.1.

Table 13.1: Key pointers away from CVD

- Sharp, electric-shock type pain – this is more likely to be neuralgia or Tietze's disease

- Reproduced by pressure – cardiac chest pain does not occur when pressure is applied

- Positional – this is more likely to be musculoskeletal or even gastric in origin

- Not related to exertion – angina is caused by the inability of the body to supply sufficient oxygen during activity

- Absence of central pain – most cardiac chest pain is central

- Continuous pain – pain that has been present for days or weeks without any respite is unlikely to be cardiac as the patient is likely to have collapsed before cardiac chest pain goes on for this long

Conditions which can mimic cardiac chest pain include pericarditis, oesophageal spasm, heartburn, pleural effusion, pulmonary embolus or even anxiety and panic attacks. It can be useful to bear in mind the following quick-fire case studies taken from my own experiences:

Martin

Martin presented with chest pain, which began two days previously. It was a sharp, electric-shock type pain which was worse when I pressed on a trigger point in the area where the pain was worse. Martin's diagnosis was Tietze's disease, otherwise known as costo-chondritis.

Leigh

Leigh presented with chest pain which had come on when he was moving furniture. It was worse when he twisted to the left. He had no other sign or symptoms. Leigh's diagnosis was a musculoskeletal strain.

Samantha

Samantha had central chest pain which was worse at night. She had also developed a cough. All investigations were normal and she was diagnosed as having reflux. Her pain and cough resolved after treatment with a proton pump inhibitor.

Abigail

Abigail was diagnosed with oesophageal spasm as her pain was not related to exertion, does not radiate, was worse lying flat or after meals and was relieved by antacids, PPIs or eructation. Confusingly, however, oesophageal spasm also responds to GTN spray!

Marion

Marion complained of sudden onset of sharp chest pain, which was worse on inspiration or lying flat. She also had a pyrexia of 38.6. She was admitted to hospital where a pericardial rub was heard and a diagnosis of viral pericarditis was made.

Wayne

Wayne was complaining of a pain in his chest accompanied by a productive cough which was worse on inspiration. Auscultation revealed the creaking gate sound of a pleural rub, typically heard in pleurisy. Further investigations revealed a lung abscess as the underlying cause.

Colin

Colin collapsed at home after complaining of severe back pain, radiating through to his abdomen, hips and thighs. He was diagnosed as having a dissecting aortic aneurysm and only his proximity to the local hospital and the swift action of his wife and the surgical team resulted in him surviving. Abdominal aortic aneurysm screening is now being carried out in some areas of the UK.

Beth

Beth came to surgery with a two-day history of left-sided chest pain and breathlessness. She was in great discomfort but examination only revealed the obvious dyspnoea and a tachycardia of 124 bpm. In view of her distress she was admitted to hospital as an emergency where a pulmonary embolism was diagnosed.

Clare

Clare, age 6, presented with chest and abdominal pain. Her temperature was 40.3, pulse 113 bpm and respiratory rate 42. She was lethargic and had not eaten or had anything to drink for 12 hours. Clare had pneumonia.

Adam

Adam, aged 12, presented with a 24-hour history of intermittent left sided chest pain. He was apyrexial and did not have a cough. He was unable to breathe in deeply due to the pain. He could not lie flat because of the pain. He had been given ibuprofen to help with the pain the night before. Auscultation revealed reduced air entry on the left. Adam was admitted where a chest X-ray revealed a mass, confirmed by scan as a benign tumour, probably present from birth and which appeared to have increased in size with puberty. He made a full recovery after excision.

Most clinicians will have a story to tell of the patient who presented with one of these unusual symptoms and it did turn out to be cardiac. The reason we remember these patients is precisely because they are not 'text book cases' and have presented in an atypical way. Nonetheless it is worth remembering that these cases do happen occasionally, just to confound us!

Remember: a good history will point you in the right direction for a correct diagnosis.

Chapter 14

Understanding chronic kidney disease

Chronic kidney disease (CKD) has a high mortality rate once it reaches the most severe stage. However, if it is diagnosed and treated earlier, then complications can be reduced and even prevented. Unfortunately, many people who develop CKD only become symptomatic when the disease is well established and at this point the opportunity for some of the interventions aimed at minimising the impact of the disease has passed. It has been said that the label of chronic kidney disease is not helpful and that rather than seeing this condition as a disease process in itself, it should be seen primarily as a risk factor for cardiovascular disease and a 'call to arms' to treat this and other CVD risk factors effectively. Nurses working in general practice are well placed to recognise people at highest risk of CKD, diagnose them and ensure that treatment is initiated and optimised in order to protect the renal and cardiovascular health of their patients in the future.

Healthy kidneys

The kidneys are two fist sized organs situated in the back, under the ribs. The role of the kidneys is to:

+ Filter the blood

+ Remove waste products

+ Return useful substances back to the body

+ Release three key hormones – erythropoietin, renin and calcitriol

Filtration of the blood is carried out by the nephrons; there are a million of these in each kidney. Each nephron consists of a tiny blood vessel, known as a glomerulus, which twists around a small tube used to collect the urine, known as a tubule. As the kidneys filter out the waste they also return protein and chemicals such as sodium, potassium and phosphate back to the body in order to maintain a healthy chemical balance.

If kidney function is significantly impaired then the ability of the kidneys to secrete hormones is also affected.

Erythropoietin (EPO) has an important role in stimulating the bone marrow to manufacture red blood cells. This is why people with severe kidney disease often suffer from anaemia. This can be treated by replacing EPO.

Renin, which is released by the nephrons in the kidneys, is important in triggering the release of angiotensin II, a powerful vasoconstrictor which maintains blood pressure and supports the circulation throughout the cardiovascular system.

Calcitriol from the kidneys is the active form of vitamin D, which is needed for bone development and to maintain a healthy chemical balance.

Impaired kidney function

Impaired kidney function is the result of damage to the filtering capacity of the nephrons. It is perfectly possible to remain quite well with only one kidney, as demonstrated when healthy family members are allowed to donate a kidney to a relative with kidney disease. In fact, it is only when kidney function drops to below a third of full function that the symptoms of renal failure may become evident.

Acute renal problems may occur in people who have ingested substances which are toxic to the kidneys, or in those who have suffered acute trauma such as a blow to the kidney. However, if acute renal failure occurs in these circumstances, the kidneys are often able to make a full recovery. Unfortunately, though, chronic kidney disease is slow to develop which means that it goes undetected until the individual becomes symptomatic or is picked up opportunistically.

Causes of CKD

There is often an associated cause for chronic kidney disease, such as hypertension and diabetes. In men, prostate disease may be another underlying cause of CKD. Clinicians should always be on the alert, too, for drugs which may impair kidney function – notably the non-steroidal anti-inflammatory drugs (NSAIDs) such as ibuprofen and diclofenac.

In terms of the link between kidney disease and hypertension, it is a bit of a chicken and egg situation. High blood pressure puts extra strain on the kidneys, leading to kidney damage. On the other hand, damaged kidneys are unable to carry out their role in maintaining a healthy blood pressure level and therefore hypertension is more likely. For this reason, tight blood pressure control is considered to be vital in protecting the kidneys in the long term. A target reading of below 140/90 (130/80 in people with diabetes and CKD) is ideal, although it is not always attainable.

Risk factors for CKD

These look remarkably similar to risk factors for CVD – a fact which underlines the importance of regarding CKD as an 'arm' of CVD. They include:

- Smoking
- Hypertension
- Diabetes
- Black or Asian ethnicity
- Existing CVD
- Long-term use of NSAIDs
- Proteinuria
- Urinary outflow tract obstruction

Signs and symptoms of kidney disease

As previously mentioned, renal impairment is often discovered during routine monitoring of blood tests for other conditions such as diabetes or hypertension. However, if this does not happen, the symptoms which are associated with renal disease include changes in the frequency of passing urine (more often, less often, new episodes of nocturia or increased frequency of nocturia), feeling tired and/or confused, poor appetite, nausea or even vomiting, oedema of the feet or hands, muscle cramps. These symptoms are attributable to the build up of waste products in the body and concurrent electrolyte imbalance.

Diagnosing kidney disease

Blood tests in a nutshell:

Testing for kidney disease – the renal Olympics:

- **Qualifying round:** a raised creatinine

- **Bronze standard:** abnormal eGFR

- **Silver standard:** Presence of microalbuminuria

- **Gold standard:** Abnormal urinary albumin:creatinine ratio

Creatinine

Creatinine is a by-product of the normal breakdown of muscle cells. In good health, the kidneys will remove creatinine from blood and excrete it via the urine. If kidney function is impaired, then creatinine levels in the blood will rise. This may be the first sign of renal disease. Unfortunately, however, creatinine levels vary enormously from person to person depending on their health status, diet, activity levels and the amount of muscle tissue in their body. For this reason, creatinine is not specific enough as a marker of renal impairment. Also, creatinine levels are not useful in diagnosing early kidney disease as a rise in creatinine only tends to occur once significant damage has occurred to the nephrons. Nonetheless, a raised creatinine level is certainly suggestive of renal disease.

GFR and eGFR

Glomerular Filtration Rate (GFR) is a measure of how effectively the kidneys are filtering waste from the bloodstream. Getting an absolute GFR for an individual patient is only possible by injecting an isotope and measuring the rate at which it is excreted. However, it is possible to get an estimated GFR (eGFR) based on the patient's creatinine measurement and using their age, gender and race to 'fine tune' an estimation of the GFR. These days most laboratories will automatically report the eGFR when a creatinine value is requested on a blood form. A simple way to think about eGFR is that the number reported relates the percentage of normal kidney function left.

Urine tests: microalbuminuria and proteinuria

Healthy kidneys remove waste products from the blood but leave protein behind as it can still be used by the body. In kidney disease, proteins are gradually able to leak through the kidneys into the urine. Albumin is a small, simple protein and is the first protein to be leaked from the kidneys in early renal disease. Testing for microalbuminuria, then, involves identifying relatively small amounts of albumin in the urine. This will not be picked up on routine dipstick testing for protein as the amount of albumin is too small. The use of specific tests designed to detect microalbuminuria should therefore be used. As the damage to the kidney increases, bigger proteins are able get through the filter into the urine in increasing amounts. The presence of large amounts of albumin and other proteins is known as proteinuria. Two tests are usually needed to confirm the presence of albumin and/or protein in the urine. The presence of infection as a cause of proteinuria should be excluded.

Albumin:Creatinine ratio

Although testing for microalbuminuria can be useful, the amount can still vary from sample to sample. A more specific test for the presence of microalbumin in the urine involves calculating the ratio of urinary albumin to the amount of urinary creatinine (ACR). Similarly, it is also possible to test for the ratio of protein to creatinine (PCR). If the first test is abnormal, another test should be done one to two weeks later, using an early morning specimen of urine, which is more reliable (Witte *et al* 2009). If the second test also shows an abnormal ratio, the diagnosis of persistent microalbuminuria (or proteinuria) has been confirmed.

An ACR of over 30mg/mmol is significant in people without diabetes. In people with diabetes, where the risk is higher, an ACR of 2.5 or more in men or 3.5 or more in women, is significant as it is diagnostic of microalbuminuria

Other investigations

People with progressive or severe CKD should be offered a renal ultrasound scan. People over the age of 20 who have a family history of polycystic kidney disease may also be offered a scan.

Ageing kidneys

In people aged 70 and over, an eGFR of 40-59 is not necessarily a problem as long as there are no other associated signs or symptoms of kidney damage, such as haematuria, and as long as the eGFR remains stable over time

Kidneys under pressure – the effect of co-morbidities

People with CKD have an increased risk of cardiovascular events such as myocardial infarction and stroke. Conversely, people with hypertension and diabetes have a higher risk of CKD too. Testing for CKD is recommended, then, for all people with the following conditions:

- ◆ Diabetes
- ◆ Hypertension
- ◆ Existing cardiovascular disease, including CHD, cerebrovascular disease, peripheral artery disease and heart failure

This is something you should consider when reviewing people with these conditions as it may not always be part of the QOF requirements. An abnormal eGFR, which has been identified during routine monitoring of bloods in patients attending for management of their hypertension or coronary heart disease, needs further assessment.

Other at risk groups who should be tested include:

- People who have evidence of haematuria or proteinuria in a 'clean' specimen of urine, which has been tested opportunistically

- People with underlying renal abnormalities such as kidney stones or prostate disease (including benign disease)

- People with diseases which are known to affect various body systems such as systemic lupus erythematosus (SLE)

- People with a family history of end stage renal disease or inherited kidney conditions such as polycystic kidney disease

Protecting the kidneys

Once people have been identified with kidney disease, the primary aim is to slow down the decline in kidney function by controlling the blood pressure. Furthermore, people who have been identified as having CKD should be considered for cardiovascular risk assessment, and treatment aimed at reducing cardiovascular risk should be prescribed where appropriate. It is important to remember that risk engines based on Framingham data are known to underestimate CVD risk in people with CKD (NICE 2008a). The Qrisk engine on the other hand (**www.qrisk.org**) asks about the presence of CKD as part of the risk assessment. Angiotensin converting enzyme (ACE) inhibitors are often the first line choice to achieve blood pressure control and protect the kidneys, particularly in people with diabetes. Risk assessment should not be necessary for people with type 2 diabetes (NICE 2008b) but in exceptional cases where risk assessment is needed, a risk engine designed especially for people with diabetes should be used (**www.dtu.ox.ac.uk/index.php?maindoc=/riskengine/**). The use of statins and aspirin should also be considered along with lifestyle advice about maintaining a healthy weight through healthy eating, increasing activity levels and stopping smoking.

Case study 24: Kathy

Putting it all into practice

Kathy is 62 years old and has a long history of hypertension. In the past she was treated with bendroflumethiazide 2.5mg and her control was poor, especially as she had been reluctant to attend surgery for check-ups, preferring simply to pick up a repeat prescription, which she did for years. With the advent of the new GMS contract and QOF, however, she had found that the surgery had insisted that she came in at least once a year for blood tests and a BP check. This year she was found to have an eGFR of 49 and the practice nurse asked to see her to discuss this.

Kathy's hypertension puts her at increased risk of CKD and her eGFR confirms this risk. The NICE guidelines have an algorithm (p9 of the Quick Reference guide for Clinical Guideline 73, available from **www.nice.org.uk**) for the management of people such as Kathy, and the practice nurse follows these closely. The next step, then, is to repeat the eGFR within two weeks. The repeat test confirms the diagnosis of CKD stage 3A. Her BP today is 152/93 mm/Hg.

The nurse discusses the implications of this diagnosis with Kathy. She explains the importance of maintaining a healthy BMI by eating a nutritionally balanced diet and taking regular exercise. She reminds Kathy to keep her alcohol within recommended limits and to avoid smoking – fortunately Kathy stopped years ago. Kathy is rather worried about her diagnosis as she fears that she will end up on dialysis if her kidneys are underperforming.

The nurse explains that this is unlikely if they continue to monitor and act upon any predisposing factors to deterioration such as poorly controlled BP. She arranges for Kathy to provide an early morning specimen of urine to assess the albumin:creatinine ratio. This is reported as being 45mg/mmol, confirmed on a second test two weeks later, and in the absence of any haematuria on dipstick testing, the nurse feels happy to manage Kathy in the surgery with the support of the GPs as necessary. Kathy will need to have an ACE inhibitor added into her current treatment, bendroflumethiazide. The nurse also explains that the biggest risk to Kathy is in terms of her cardiovascular health and that this will be addressed by starting her on a statin. Kathy uses ibuprofen for her osteoarthritis and the nurse explains how this may be contributing to her renal problems. Kathy decides to switch to paracetamol with some codeine added in if the pain is not well controlled.

Case study 25: Danny

Danny, age 58, has recently been diagnosed with type 2 diabetes and has been confirmed as having CKD stage 3B. His BP is 142/91. The treatment plan for his CKD will follow a similar path to Kathy's, in that an ACE inhibitor will be advisable to control his BP. An ACE such as ramipril will be initiated at a low dose (1.25-2.5mg daily) and renal function will be monitored closely after 10-14 days. If renal function remains stable then the ACE will be uptitrated to 10mg over a period of weeks with renal function tests being repeated after each dose increase. A fall in eGFR of less than 25% is considered acceptable (NICE 2008a) but regular monitoring will be needed to ensure that renal function stabilises and is not progressively deteriorating. If eGFR falls by 25% or more, or potassium levels rise to 6mmol/L or more, further advice should be sought, as the ACE may need to be stopped. Care should be taken with serum potassium levels above 5mmol/L as a further rise may follow. Danny's target BP will be below 130/80 as his risk of complications is higher due his diabetes. The clinical knowledge summaries website (**www.cks.library.nhs.uk/home**) includes examples of how to initiate and uptitrate ACE inhibitors in CKD. If Danny is unable to tolerate an ACE due to cough, an angiotensin receptor blocker such as irbesartan or olmesartan may be used instead. Metformin may not be an option for treating his diabetes as this is contraindicated in renal impairment due to the risk of lactic acidosis (**www.bnf.org**) and he may need a sulphonylurea, a post-prandial insulin secretagogue (e.g. repaglinide) or insulin to treat his blood glucose levels.

Table 14.1: Action plans based on stages of CKD

Stage 1 - eGFR: 90+

Meaning: These people have apparently good renal function of 90% or more but have other evidence of kidney damage, e.g. proteinuria or haematuria

Key Action: Manage CVD risk factors including BP, lipids, weight and smoking

Repeat eGFR: Annually

Stage 2 - eGFR: 60-89

Meaning: Renal function is only slightly impaired at 60-89% but there is other evidence of kidney damage as above

Key Action: Manage CVD risk factors as above

Repeat eGFR: Annually

Stage 3a - eGFR: 45-59

Meaning: Renal function is moderately impaired at 45-59%. There may be other evidence of kidney damage

Key Action: Manage CVD risk factors as above

Repeat eGFR: 6 monthly

Stage 3b - eGFR: 30-44

Meaning: As above

Key Action: Manage CVD risk factors as above. Risk of renal anaemia increases. Monitor Hb and treat if <11g/dl, excluding other causes of anaemia first

Repeat eGFR: 6 monthly

Table 14.1: Action plans based on stages of CKD

Stage 4 - eGFR: 15-29

Meaning: Renal function is severely impaired at 15-29%

Key Action: Should be seen by renal specialist. Manage CVD risk factors. Identify and manage bone conditions. Monitor Hb and treat if <11g/dl

Repeat eGFR: 3 monthly

Stage 5 - eGFR: <15

Meaning: Established renal failure

Key Action: Should be seen by renal specialist. Manage CVD risk factors. Identify and manage bone conditions. Monitor Hb and treat if <11g/dl

Repeat eGFR: 6 weekly

Other key considerations when managing people with CKD:

- Involve people in decisions about their care

- Try to personalise information to the individual, taking account of the stage of CKD that they have, their support network and their own needs, both physical and psychological

- Stress the importance of a healthy lifestyle in optimising both cardiovascular and renal health – diet, weight, exercise, smoking cessation, BP control and lipid management

- Routine dietary restriction of protein is no longer recommended but salt restriction should be implemented in all patients, in line with healthy eating advice

- Discourage the use of NSAIDs

- Recommend flu and pneumonia jabs

Bone health

- Routine blood tests for bone health (serum calcium, phosphate and parathyroid hormone) are not recommended for CKD 1-3

- People with CKD stage 1-3 who are thought to be at risk of osteoporosis because of other risk factors (family history, smoking, lack of exercise) may be offered treatment with a bisphosphonate

- Vitamin D supplements (cholecalciferol or ergocalciferol) may also be required

When to refer

- CKD stage 4 and 5

- People with ACR results of 70mg/mmol unless they are known to have diabetes and are on an ACE inhibitor (ARB if unable to tolerate an ACE) at the maximum tolerated dose

- People with an ACR of >30mg/mmol plus haematuria

- People whose eGFR is declining rapidly (defined as a decrease of >5ml per year or >10ml within five years)

- People with poorly controlled blood pressure in spite of treatment with four drugs as per the BHS/NICE guidelines (NICE 2006)

- People with rare causes of CKD or possible renal artery stenosis

The referral letter should contain information about previous renal function tests as well as the latest, past medical history, current drug therapy and blood tests.

Shared care may well be possible between the GP practice and the specialist once a care plan has been established and agreed. Clinicians will need to take particular note of advice on treatment surrounding EPO replacement therapy and the use of calcitriol in terms of specific indications for monitoring these patients.

In summary then, CKD is common, occurring in 1 in 10 of the population, although very few of these will need dialysis. It is a strong marker for CVD risk and treatment of CVD risk factors, using both pharmacological and lifestyle approaches is vital. The use of blood and urine tests to monitor renal function is important as it will allow clinicians to identify those at risk of complications and to initiate treatment which will reduce the risk of further deterioration. Nurses working in general practice should be aware of the risk of CVD in patients with other long term conditions and should ensure that screening and identification is carried out.

References

Cox, Beverley. Improving the Care of Patients with Chronic Kidney Disease.
British Journal of Primary Care Nursing – Cardiovascular Disease and Diabetes, Volume 6, Issue 2 April-June 2009 Pages 8-11. www.bjpcn-cardiovascular.com

Witte E et al (2009). First morning voids are more reliable than spot urine samples to assess microalbuminuria. Journal of the American Society of Nephrology 20(2):436-43

Resources

Clinical Knowledge Summaries: Guidelines on managing CKD available from: *www.cks.library.nhs.uk/home*

NICE (2006) Clinical Guideline 34; Hypertension available from: *www.nice.org.uk/nicemedia/pdf/cg034quickrefguide.pdf*

NICE (2008a) Clinical Guideline 73; Chronic Kidney Disease available from: *www.nice.org.uk/Guidance/CG73*

NICE (2008b) Clinical Guideline 66 Type 2 diabetes: the management of type 2 diabetes (update) available from: *www.nice.org.uk/Guidance/CG66*

NSF for Renal Services (2004 and 2005) available from: *www.dh.gov.uk*

Resources for patients

www.renal.org.uk

www.bhf.org.uk

www.diabetes.org.uk

www.kidney.org.uk

www.patient.co.uk

www.nhs.uk/Pathways/Kidneydisease/Pages/Landing.aspx

The importance of ensuring a successful therapeutic alliance in the secondary prevention of CVD in high risk patients

Case study 26: Hamish

Hamish, age 53, rarely attends surgery as he is 'simply too busy'. He came in two years ago asking whether he could get Viagra on prescription but other than that has not been seen. At the time, the nurse, Marianne, did manage to get him to agree to have a BP check and also gave him a form for a blood test for lipids and blood glucose but he did not attend. Marianne had noticed that he could be at risk of metabolic syndrome as he had a big tummy and a BP of 149/93.

The next time Marianne saw Hamish he was attending the coronary heart disease clinic, having recently been diagnosed with acute coronary syndrome. This came as a great shock to him as he is a self-employed businessman and had always thrived on the cut-and-thrust atmosphere of selling insurance. One morning, whilst preparing for an important business meeting he noticed that he was getting indigestion-type pains which he put down to the restaurant curry and three pints of beer that he had the night before. Over the next hour, however, the pain became worse and started to form a tight band around his chest and he also began to feel nauseous, clammy and generally quite unwell. His usual antacids were not helping at all so as his surgery offered a same-day appointment service he decided to pop in and get some stronger antacids before his meeting began.

When he arrived at the surgery, the receptionist immediately realised that Hamish was very ill and an ambulance was summoned on a 999 call. Hamish was diagnosed with a non-ST elevation myocardial infarction (non-STEMI). During his in-patient stay he was also found to have undiagnosed type 2 diabetes.

After completing a course of cardiac rehabilitation, Hamish attended the surgery for follow-up and ongoing care. A review of his medication was carried out. His current therapy included ramipril 10mg, carvedilol 25mg bd, metformin 500mg bd, aspirin 75mg and a high intensity statin in line with NICE guidance for patients who have suffered acute coronary syndrome. Hamish was not impressed with having to take all of these tablets and wanted to know 'which ones he could come off first'. It took some time to explain to Hamish that this was not a course of treatment but that these drugs needed to be taken for life in order to protect his heart and reduce the risk of a further event.

Hamish was reviewed again three months later after having blood tests repeated to assess his current status. He had recently returned to work and was feeling much better for this. His HbA1c, at 8.2% was above the recommended level of <7%, but his BP was acceptable at 129/81. Clearly more work would be needed regarding control of his diabetes and Marianne decided to increase his metformin from 500mg bd to 1g bd. She also noticed that his lipid profile remained abnormal with a total cholesterol of 6.8mmol, an HDL of 0.9mmol and triglycerides of 2mmol. Further discussion with Hamish revealed that he was not actually taking his statin. The reason, he said, was that he had suffered from aching all over after he started on all of his treatment and after reading an article in his daily newspaper, had decided that the statin was to blame. He had stopped it immediately and had started to feel better about 10 days later.

Marianne explained that although muscle aches could be a side effect of statins, it could also be that Hamish was simply feeling the after effects of his recent episode of ill-health. Even if the statin was to blame, the chances were that the side effects could wear off as time went on. Hamish agreed, albeit reluctantly, to give it another try. Two days later he was back, complaining vociferously that the pains were back. Marianne arranged blood tests, including creatine kinase, to see whether Hamish was suffering from the rare but potentially fatal side effect known as rhabdomyolysis. The blood tests actually came back within normal limits but Hamish was adamant that he would not take another statin. Marianne then had to consider other possible options.

NICE guidance recommends that there are other options available for patients who are unable to tolerate a statin. These include ezetimibe, fibrates, bile acid sequestrants and nicotinic acid. Ezetimibe is a treatment used to lower lipid levels in two ways. Firstly, it prevents cholesterol which has been produced in the liver then released via the bile duct into the intestine from being reabsorbed into the bloodstream. Secondly, it reduces the amount of cholesterol from dietary sources being absorbed from the small intestine. Ezetimibe is normally used in combination with a statin tablet. When used together they can have a more powerful cholesterol lowering effect. Ezetimibe can be used alone, though, if someone is unable to take a statin for any reason. The recommended dose of ezetimibe is one 10mg tablet a day. Ezetimibe is generally well tolerated.

There is some evidence that fibrates can reduce the risk of CVD and can impact on HDL and triglyceride levels in particular, and that they may be useful for people who require supplementary treatment after statin therapy or for those who cannot tolerate statin treatment at all in secondary prevention.

Nicotinic acid has been shown to reduce LDL-C and triglycerides and increase HDL-C but is not well tolerated due to a range of side effects, including facial flushing. Nicotinic acid may be prescribed as a slow release tablet to reduce side effects. A new version of nicotinic acid therapy became available in 2008, which combines nicotinic acid with an anti-flushing agent (laropiprant). Nicotinic acid should normally be used with a statin but can be used alone for people who cannot tolerate a statin.

Bile acid sequestrants remove bile acids from the body; this makes the body respond by converting cholesterol in the blood to bile acids to try to stabilise levels. This results in reduced blood cholesterol levels. There is insufficient evidence that these drugs (e.g. cholestyramine) can be recommended routinely in lipid management unless people cannot tolerate statins. Bile acid sequestrants are associated with a high incidence of gastro-intestinal side effects for some individuals, the main side effect being constipation.

Marianne explained all of this to Hamish and he decided that he would prefer to take ezetimibe as he felt that he would 'always get any side effect going'. In the interests of ensuring a successful therapeutic alliance with the patient, Marianne agreed that ezetimibe was a reasonable choice and arranged for him to have a prescription and for further blood tests to be carried out in another six weeks.

Negotiation, involving patients in decision making about their treatment, and ensuring that consent has been obtained correctly to take or refuse treatment, is a vital part of the health professional's role. The media often report stories on cardio-vascular disease, risk factors and treatment for dyslipidaemia which may be widely misleading. It is important that health professionals are able to hear and respect the point of view of the patient and to interact in a way that allows clear understanding between the individuals concerned. A thorough knowledge of the evidence behind lipid disorders and the lifestyle and drug interventions that can be used is vital. NICE stress the importance of patient-centred care when treating dyslipidaemia and its associated increase in CVD.

Patient Centred Care

Healthcare professionals should use every-day, jargon-free language when discussing CVD risk, lifestyle modifications and treatments with patients. Adequate time should be set aside for the consultation to allow questions to be answered, and further consultation may be needed. Discussions with patients about CVD risk should be documented. Treatment and care should take into account:

◆ a person's needs and preferences

◆ a person's culture and any physical, sensory or learning disabilities

◆ the need to ensure effective communication of information if a person does not speak or read English, as their first language

If the patient agrees, families and carers should have the opportunity to be involved in decisions about treatment and care.

Amended from the NICE Lipid Modification guidelines (2008)

Index